MASTERING
KEMPO

William Durbin

Soke

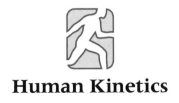

Human Kinetics

Library of Congress Cataloging-in-Publication Data

Durbin, William, 1953-
    Mastering Kempo / William Durbin
        p.   cm.
    Includes index.
    ISBN 0-7360-0350-9
        1. Kung fu. I. Title.

    GV1114.D87   2001
    796.815'.9--dc21

                                                                                    00-061340

ISBN: 0-7360-0350-9

Assistant Editor: Wendy McLaughlin; **Copyeditor:** Robert Replinger; **Proofreader:** Myla Smith; **Indexer:** Sharon Duffy; **Graphic Designer:** Robert Reuther; **Graphic Artist:** Francine Hamerski; **Photo Manager:** Clark Brooks; **Cover Designer:** Keith Blomberg; **Photographer (cover and interior):** Tom Roberts; **Printer:** United Graphics

Human Kinetics books are available at special discounts for bulk purchase. Special editions or book excerpts can also be created to specification. For details, contact the Special Sales Manager at Human Kinetics.

Printed in the United States of America   10   9   8   7   6   5   4   3   2   1

Human Kinetics
Web site: www.humankinetics.com

United States: Human Kinetics
P.O. Box 5076
Champaign, IL 61825-5076
800-747-4457
e-mail: humank@hkusa.com

Canada: Human Kinetics
475 Devonshire Road Unit 100
Windsor, ON N8Y 2L5
800-465-7301 (in Canada only)
e-mail: hkcan@mnsi.net

Europe: Human Kinetics
P.O. Box IW14
Leeds LS16 6TR, United Kingdom
+44 (0) 113 278 1708
e-mail: humank@hkeurope.com

Australia: Human Kinetics
57A Price Avenue
Lower Mitcham, South Australia 5062
08 82771555
e-mail: liahka@senet.com.au

New Zealand: Human Kinetics
P.O. Box 105-231
Auckland Central
09-309-1890
e-mail: hkp@ihug.co.nz

For my parents, the late Mr. and Mrs. William Durbin

Without their encouragement I could not have become the person I am today. They taught me to believe in God, love unconditionally, and gave me my start in the martial arts.

CONTENTS

FOREWORD

It is with great pleasure that I recommend *Mastering Kempo* to the public. I began my association with William Durbin in 1978 when he attended a clinic I was giving in Cincinnati. I found him a personable individual with a remarkable dedication to the martial arts. At that time, I was living in Memphis, Tennessee. Bill began traveling there to train with me and joined me at clinics throughout the States.

Over the years I have watched Bill progress in his command and knowledge of the martial arts, especially Kempo. Having taught for Elvis Presley at the Tennessee Karate Institute, I was exposed to many Kempo practitioners over the years, especially those from the International Kenpo Karate Association of Ed Parker, and I understand the intricacies of this marvelous martial art.

Bill is one of the leading practitioners of Kempo, with an in-depth knowledge of the history and philosophy of the martial arts. In *Mastering Kempo,* Bill reveals little-known information that will be of interest to all Kempo practitioners, as well as martial artists of other styles. I recommend this book heartily to all martial artists who wish to expand their knowledge and understanding of the intricacies of the martial arts.

Bill "Superfoot" Wallace

PREFACE

Kempo, one of the most effective self-defense martial arts ever to come out of the Orient, first came to the United States in 1942. Over the years it has spread throughout the country, and from there the world.

Although Kempo is taught in most countries of the world, many misconceptions and misunderstandings have developed because of a lack of historical perspective and vague documentation.

The main difference between fighting arts and what came to be called martial arts is the attitude toward peace. Fighting arts were designed to defeat an enemy, usually with the idea of killing him. As sporting events, fighting arts were brutal, ending in the severe injury or death of one of the participants.

Martial arts were not about killing or competition, but about survival and harmony. In ancient times, martial-arts competitions like those we see today did not exist. Instead, martial arts used methods of training that required the harmonious interaction of training partners to achieve the greatest development of skill.

The ultimate goal of martial-arts training was to survive conflict, without fighting when possible. When combat was unavoidable, the practitioner did no more than necessary to end a confrontation. This is the heart of Kempo, the original martial art.

Mastering Kempo shows the basic techniques common to all methods of Kempo, as well as advanced skills and ways of combining them to develop mastery of the art. *Mastering Kempo* is an attempt to explain Kempo as it was transmitted to the United States and around the world. More important, it is an exposition of Kempo as the masters originally taught it. The book includes their methods of training, which many have ignored in modern times. *Mastering Kempo* will introduce you to techniques, skills, and advanced methods that will enrich the Kempo of any stylist and contribute to an in-depth understanding of the many martial arts derived from Kempo, which include Judo, Jujutsu, and Karate.

May this book enrich your philosophy, expand your mind, and give you the technical skills to enhance your training.

ACKNOWLEDGMENTS

I gratefully acknowledge my personal instructors in Kempo, Richard Stone, Bill "Superfoot" Wallace, and Dr. Rod Sacharnoski for setting such a good example in training and humility. I am thankful for their spiritual support, mental instruction, and technical training.

Also, I want to recognize all of the students of Kiyojute Ryu for their support and participation in the family of "spiritually positive, gentle people." Most especially I thank my wife for the freedom and support as I fill my life with Kempo.

Finally, thank you to all the wonderful people at Human Kinetics who helped me achieve my goal of getting this book published.

The History and Influence of Kempo

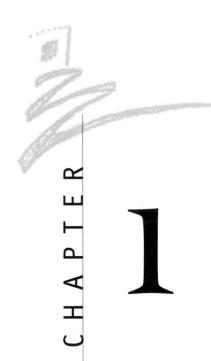

Since the beginning of time, humankind has used various forms of fighting. Families and clans developed skills and abilities in combat, and they passed on the methods that proved successful. Eventually, a level of enlightenment developed within humanity. Enlightenment can be understood as seeing the light that is beyond the phenomenal world. This is the goal of all religious faiths, seeing into the ultimate or experiencing oneness with the light. People who were not interested in fighting but who understood the need for self-defense began to formulate methods dedicated to peace rather than fighting.

The ultimate goal of martial-arts training was to survive conflict without fighting whenever possible. When combat was unavoidable, a person did no more to end a confrontation than necessary. This concept is the heart of Kempo, the original martial art.

THE LEGEND OF BODHIDHARMA (CHINA)

According to legend, martial arts started in the sixth century with the religious personage Bodhidharma. He was born in India to a family of the Kshatriya, the warrior caste. As such, he would have been trained in the fighting art known as Vajramushti, which means the "diamond fist."

He traveled from his home in India to China, where he wanted to teach his religion. When he arrived in China, however, he found that Buddhism had become materialistic, focusing on deeds rather than experience. The Chinese Buddhist believers had become enamored of building elaborate temples, making statues, and translating scriptures. The inner changes that come with the experience of enlightenment were absent. Frustrated by the ruling class, he traveled to the Shaolin monastery. He meditated there for nine years before deciding to teach the monks, who showed interest in and worthiness for his teachings. Bodhidharma taught a unique form of meditation that became known as Chan, which in Japanese is pronounced Zen. This meditation focuses on experiencing oneness rather than believing in doctrines.

As he began teaching, Bodhidharma found the monks at the temple in poor physical health with little endurance for meditation. They could not even stay awake during his sermons. Thus he created a series of exercises from Vajramushti, which became known as Shih Pa Lo Han Sho, or the "18 hands of an enlightened man."

He saw that the monks and villagers, who depended on the temple for religious guidance, were at the mercy of bandits and brigands who roamed the hills taking what they wanted. Therefore, he taught the monks how to use the movements of the exercises in a combative manner.

But he would not compromise the pacifistic nature of his faith. He explained to the monks that this method of combat must be Wu, based on stopping violence. It was to be a matter of Wute, or peaceful virtue. The term Wu, pronounced Bu in Japanese, is now translated as "martial," but the real meaning is "to stop violence." Te is pronounced Toku, thus Wute is known as Butoku in Japanese. Therefore, we can see that the first and original martial art, Wu Shu, or Bujutsu in Japanese, was based on a combination of excellent fighting skill and religious virtue.

It is believed that the monks named the new art after a combination of Dharma, which is the "truth of Buddhism," and Mushti, which is "fist." In Chinese, Dharma is Ho, while Mushti is Chuan. Thus the art was called Chuanfa, the law of the fist. In Japanese, this is pronounced Kempo.

As the Shaolin monks began to defeat opponents with exceptional skill, their fighting prowess quickly reached legendary proportions. It is reported that a group of monks once fought off 10 times their number in a battle against Mongol invaders.

As the fame of Shaolinssu Chuanfa, referred to hereafter by its Japanese pronunciation Shorinji Kempo, diffused through China, many others sought to practice the martial art. As other temples adopted the fighting method, the skill spread throughout China. Some monks started teaching their lay charges, and secular variations of the art began to develop.

NAKANO (JAPAN)

Originally, Shorinji Kempo was primarily a fist and palm art. It was preserved that way in at least one style, according to Michiomi Nakano, the first So Doshin of Nippon Shorinji Kempo, a Japanese variation that developed at the end of World War II. Nakano (who started using the title, So Doshin, as his name) was the man most responsible for preserving many ancient methods of training, which have nearly been lost with the development of modern sport forms of martial arts.

Nakano taught that Kempo was actually the other half of religious training at the Shaolin temple. Zen was the static form of meditation, whereas Kempo was the active form. Zen was the stillness; Kempo was the motion. In stillness the monks sought motion; in motion they sought stillness. To achieve full enlightenment, it was believed that one must use both forms of training. In particular, Kempo helped people manifest their insights in real life, just as they trained to stay calm and peaceful while engaged in martial-arts training and actual combat.

THE BUDDHISTS (KOREA, JAPAN, OKINAWA)

During the 6th, 12th, and 17th centuries, the Buddhists staged evangelical movements by which they sought to spread their faith throughout the Orient. Their religions reached Korea, Japan, and Okinawa, as did their form of Kempo, which influenced development of the indigenous fighting arts and helped them evolve into true martial arts.

In the Japanese language, Chinese Chuanfa is pronounced Chugoku Kempo, literally the "middle kingdom fist law." According to James Masayoshi Mitose, the headmaster of Kosho Ryu Kempo, Chugoku Kempo brought a depth of philosophical and technical proficiency to the indigenous fighting arts that was not known before.

During the 6th century and especially during the 12th century, the martial arts developed markedly in Japan and Okinawa. The people in the temples and rural areas continued to develop their martial arts, but it was the influence of Kempo in these two periods that brought about the greatest changes. Sohei were warrior monks who protected the temples from bandits and corrupt government officials. They were highly skilled in the martial arts and even helped the rural Samurai develop their skills.

Under the influence of Chugoku Kempo, monks in the temples of Japan and Okinawa developed distinctive forms of Kempo adapted to their environment and culture, particularly their customs of warfare. In the warm climate of Okinawa, where the people wore much less clothing and used little armor, the Kempo centered on the use of the fist and other empty-hand striking skills. Although the royalty kept swords and other weapons for the defense of the nation, especially against the Wako, pirates who plied the waters around the islands, commoners primarily used Chugoku Kempo for protection, though they did learn to use their tools as weapons.

According to Kenichi Sawai, when Chugoku Kempo came to Japan, people realized that the training was something special. In Japan, the Chugoku Kempo became known as Shinken, or divine fists, meaning "divinely inspired martial arts." These were seen as distinctly different from mere fighting arts, which had only the defeat of the enemy in mind. These true martial arts were concerned with the development of peace and harmony for all humankind.

In the 16th century, the generic term Jujutsu was coined for all empty-hand combat forms in Japan. But several of the Ryu, systems of martial arts that began developing during the 12th century, maintained the use of the term Kempo or maintained a branch of their Jujutsu art specifically dealing with Kempo. A few styles, most prominently Kosho Ryu, combined the new name with the older one to form the phrase Kempo Jujutsu.

OKINAWA

In Okinawa, the indigenous art was known as Te, meaning "hand" but referring to skill. When the Chinese influence arrived, Kempo became a common term used to express the martial arts. Eventually other prefixes were applied to Te, so that terms such as Karate, Bushite, and others were coined. In modern times the term Karate is the most common name for Okinawan martial arts. Karate means "empty hand" and refers to the philosophical concept of emptiness rather than a lack of weaponry.

Several styles of Okinawan martial arts prefer to use the term Kempo Karate to give a more complete interpretation of the style, showing the connection to the old while keeping the philosophical meaning of empty hand. Later, I will explain more about the relationship of modern Jujutsu and Karate to their source art, Kempo.

STYLES OF MARTIAL ARTS

Five styles of martial arts were developed, including Shinken, Himitsu, Gogyo, Heiho, and Kamite.

Shinken

The Japanese coined the term Shinken for a type of martial art. Shin is the Japanese term that can be translated as "God," "soul," "venerable," "hallowed," or "divine." Ken, the term for fist, is used generically in China and sometimes in Japan to mean "martial art" or, in the most esoteric sense, "unified man."

Thus the term Shinken was used for a martial art that was divinely inspired. The inspiration could have come from the soul of the person or from God on high. In the Japanese Shinto concept, Shin could also mean "a divine being," like an angel. In Japan this could also be a Tengu, a goblinlike angel, which was said to have inspired several martial artists in later Japanese history.

The divine fist of the Chinese martial arts became the inspiration for many of the martial arts of both Japan and Okinawa. But more important, it became a process of personal development. The warriors of both Japan and Okinawa began to seek a spiritual basis for their fighting skill. All warriors, at least those who achieved any renown, used prayer and meditation to seek inspiration from a divine source for the development of their martial art.

Himitsu Kempo

Himitsu Kempo training started with a special form of instruction called Karumijutsu, which had its origin in China. This term literally means "the art of body lightening." Orientals believed that a person who had learned to be light and airy on the feet in a physical manner had achieved a level of spiritual lightness as well.

Gogyo

Certain forms of Kempo then taught the concept of Gogyo, a strategic method of combat based on the five elements. The idea was that each element could overcome another. Water, for example, could overcome fire. An element could also give rise to another. For instance, earth could generate metal.

Heiho

The Heiho of fighting strategy turned into Heiho, now written with the Kanji (characters) meaning "law of peace." Heiho helps the martial artist become a more peaceful person, a person who seeks to make a harmonious life with all others.

Kamite

In Okinawa, a level of martial-arts training referred to as Kamite was developed. According to many sources, this art formed the foundation of all branches of Karate that developed in Okinawan martial arts.

CHANGES IN KEMPO

When Kempo came to Japan and Okinawa through the Buddhist monks, it did not retain its original form for three reasons.

Culture

The first reason is cultural. Each people, each country, has a distinct attitude that determines how people respond or behave, including how they fight and react. The Chinese martial artist tended to be oriented to vengeance and thus developed skills especially suited to attack and revenge.

In Japan, on the other hand, the ruling class of Bushi, warriors who "served" the emperor while actually ruling in his stead, were obsessed with honor. They fought one to one, face to face, in "honorable," personal combat. Thus, at least initially, they developed skills for lethal dueling.

In Okinawa, the people tended to be more laid back and friendly. Little violence dwelled in the Okinawan heart. Instead, they held a real desire to live in peace and harmony. Yet they realized that violence was part of life and that they had to be able to defend themselves against an irate person, bandits, and, especially in their situation, pirates. Thus the skills they developed were almost exclusively for self-defense.

Kempo—The Proper Rendering

Much discussion has occurred about the proper way to write the word Kempo. In Japanese this word is made up of two Kanji, or Chinese characters. The first is Ken, meaning "fist," and the second is Ho, meaning "law, way, or method." Thus Kempo can be translated as "law of the fist," "fist way," or "fist method."

Regarding pronunciation, the standard for transliterating Japanese Kanji into English is the Rose-Innes method. This phonetically renders what one hears into the Romanized form. Where an *h* follows an *n*, the *n* takes on an *m* sound, and the *h* takes on a *p* sound. Thus *Ken* and *Ho* is pronounced Kempo.

Today, many people spell it Kenpo because of a typographical error made in 1953. In 1947,

James Masayoshi Mitose wrote a book titled *What Is Self-Defense? Kempo JiuJitsu*, which was finally published in 1953. But the publisher mistakenly spelled Kempo with an *n*. Lacking the funds to have the book republished, Mitose left it the way it was. His student, William Chow, used the rendering Kenpo in referring to the martial art he developed, calling it Kenpo Karate. Ed Parker kept this spelling as well, bringing it with him to the continental United States.

Both are acceptable forms of transliterating the Kanji into English, though for those who wish to be formally correct, the Rose-Innes method produces the word Kempo.

In Japan, the Kempo of the temples was comprehensive, having all the skills of combat. Temple Kempo contained throws, joint locks, holds, chokes, blocks, strikes, thrusts, kicks, and body blows. Originally, the temple used weapons made only of wood, such as staffs and walking sticks. As the temples came into conflict with government warriors, they found it necessary to learn the use of the traditional weapons of war—Katana (swords), Yari (spears), and Naginata (halberds).

Combat Application

The monks also taught their Kempo to the Samurai who supported their temples and religion. This led to the second reason the martial arts changed—the difference in combat application. The Samurai would have been of two general categories (though this is a simplification of a complex system of government). The Bushi were the high-level Samurai. They generally fought in heavy armor and thus used empty-hand techniques suited to fighting men similarly armed. It would be impossible to pick up a person in heavy armor in hip throws or shoulder wheels, or to produce an effective strike against a person who had vital points protected by strong armor. But attacking the wrists, elbows, and shoulders with joint locks was extremely effective. Therefore, the Bushi developed what is today called Aikijujutsu. The Bushi also developed some throws based on armor clashing. In this method, the Bushi threw their armored form against that of an opponent, knocking the enemy off balance. Through control of momentum and body position, the Bushi could hurl the enemy to the ground.

The second category of Samurai would be the Ashigaru, or foot soldiers. They generally used the Yari or Naginata as their primary weapon and backed it up with empty-hand skills based on throws that used leg reaps, foot sweeps, props, hip throws, and hand skills. These skills are generally known as Jujutsu.

Through the efforts of Jigoro Kano, Jujutsu eventually developed into the modern martial sport known as Judo, which in 1964 became an Olympic sport. In 1942, the Shinto priest Morihei Ueshiba modified Aikijujutsu into the modern spiritual discipline and excellent form of self-defense known as Aikido. These arts owe their origins to the Kempo of the Japanese temples.

In Okinawa, the ruling class had its own martial art, which was based on their cultural roots that originally came from Japan. The emperors were descendants of Tametomo Minamoto, who came to Okinawa in the 12th century. He married an Okinawan woman who bore him a son named Shunten. This young man went on to unite Okinawa under one rule and establish dynasties that lasted until the 19th century.

The ruling class of Okinawa learned from any source they could, yet they maintained the foundation of the Minamoto Bujutsu martial arts. During the 12th and 14th centuries, substantial interaction occurred between China and Okinawa. Priests, military attachés, and other Chinese martial artists brought Chugoku Kempo to the attention of the Okinawan ruling class and to a few commoners.

In general, the Okinawan martial art was called Te. The royalty used the term Bushi Te to refer to their art based on the skill of the Bushi warrior. Only members of the royalty learned this "warrior hand" martial art.

The few commoners who learned Chinese martial arts referred to their art simply as either Kempo or Tode, which can also be pronounced Karate, written with the Chinese characters meaning "Tang hand," referring to the Tang dynasty of China. This acknowledged the Chinese influence.

Modernization

The final reason for the modification of Kempo was modernization and a change in emphasis from warring art to peacetime activity. Evidence of this is seen in China itself. Tai Chi evolved into an exercise that gave up or modified many of the martial arts techniques. Wu Shu has become very much a gymnastic event, with few movements applicable to combat.

In Japan, as peace developed during the Tokugawa era from 1603 to 1868, an emphasis on prearranged forms and sporting bouts emerged. Participants used mock swords, made either of wood (Bokken) or bamboo (Shinai). An unrealistic and aggressive form of martial sport resulted. In many of these sports, the techniques no longer have application to actual combat or self-defense. When empty-hand schools followed suit, the sport of Judo developed, and under the influence of one of Morihei Ueshiba's students, a sport of Aikido emerged.

On Okinawa, the situation was different. The Okinawan masters in 1936 began calling their art Karate, meaning "empty hand," emphasizing the philosophical concept of emptiness. The masters still felt that their art of Kempo was too dangerous to play with, and thus they did not develop a sport form.

The Japanese, however, had become aware of the Okinawan martial art in the early 1900s. In the 1920s, some Okinawan masters began teaching Karate in Japan. The three main teachers were Choki Motobu, Gichin

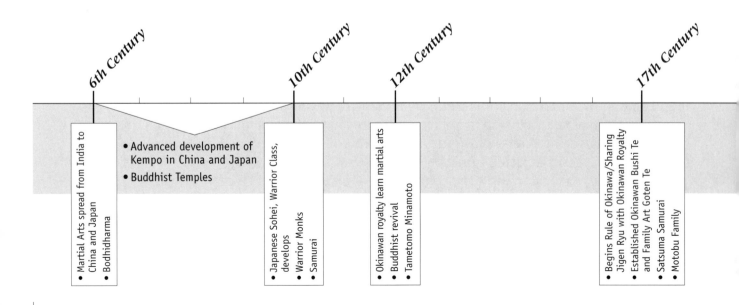

6th Century
- Martial Arts spread from India to China and Japan
- Bodhidharma

• Advanced development of Kempo in China and Japan
• Buddhist Temples

10th Century
- Japanese Sohei, Warrior Class, develops
- Warrior Monks
- Samurai

12th Century
- Okinawan royalty learn martial arts
- Buddhist revival
- Tametomo Minamoto

17th Century
- Begins Rule of Okinawa/Sharing Jigen Ryu with Okinawan Royalty
- Established Okinawan Bushi Te and Family Art Goten Te
- Satsuma Samurai
- Motobu Family

Funakoshi, and Kenwa Mabuni. Each of these masters, at one time, called their art Kempo Karate.

During this time, Japanese students, being more competitive than their Okinawan counterparts, began to try each other in sparring matches. Whereas Okinawan martial-arts teachers would have stepped in and disciplined their students, forbidding them to engage in this type of free fighting, the Japanese instructors chose to develop rules under which their students could battle each other. Thus the Karate Shiai, or contest, was born.

A few dedicated Okinawan masters still teach their martial art in the old manner and refuse to allow their students to engage in any form of sport combat. These masters generally teach in the old manner without prearranged Kata, which is another outgrowth of the modernization of the art of Karate.

In the past, an Okinawan master taught only a small number of students and thus could lead them in freestyle Kata, which allowed the students to learn their master's methods of fighting. When Okinawa started using Te as a method of physical fitness in public schools, the main teacher in charge, Yasutsune Itosu, noted how much easier it would be to teach a group of children by using prearranged sets. These prearranged Kata, which would allow easy testing, group learning, and safe training, became the standard way of teaching Karate.

This method was extremely safe because students did not learn the secrets of combat unless they were taught the process of Bunkai, the analysis of movements, from which to derive Oyo, the fighting applications of motion. Without this type of training, which instructors withheld until students were considered old enough or mature enough, the students had basically learned only how to dance. They were no threat to others or themselves.

Thus we see that Kempo is the original martial art, spread throughout the Orient by Buddhist monks. Kempo influenced the development of fighting arts into true martial arts, on both a philosophical and technical level.

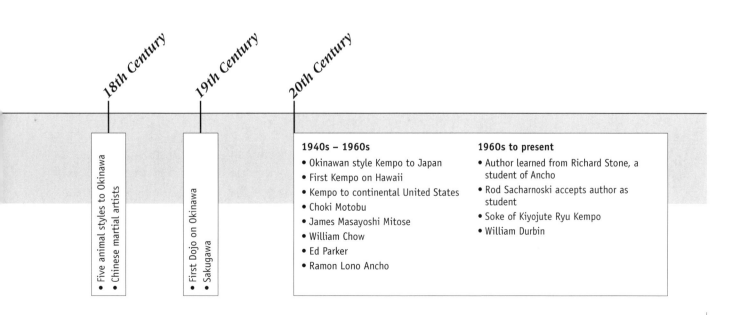

18th Century
- Five animal styles to Okinawa
- Chinese martial artists

19th Century
- First Dojo on Okinawa
- Sakugawa

20th Century

1940s – 1960s
- Okinawan style Kempo to Japan
- First Kempo on Hawaii
- Kempo to continental United States
- Choki Motobu
- James Masayoshi Mitose
- William Chow
- Ed Parker
- Ramon Lono Ancho

1960s to present
- Author learned from Richard Stone, a student of Ancho
- Rod Sacharnoski accepts author as student
- Soke of Kiyojute Ryu Kempo
- William Durbin

Because of cultural differences, contrasting methods of waging war, and eventual modernization, Kempo developed into Jujutsu in Japan, which turned into Judo and Aikido, and into Karate in Okinawa.

STYLES OF KEMPO

Both Karate and Jujutsu owe their existence to the ancient art of Kempo. Although both arts teach effective skills, they tend to be less comprehensive than the original Kempo of their countries. Pure Chugoku Kempo, Chinese martial art, lacks the inspirations found in Japan and Okinawa.

The most complete system of Kempo is that of Okinawa simply because Okinawa was a melting pot for the martial arts of Japan and China and contained the unique genius of the Okinawan warriors themselves. The Bushi of Okinawa began with the Minamoto Bujutsu, as noted earlier, brought to their island by Tametomo Minamoto.

This style would have included not only typical Japanese weapon skills but also, and more important, the empty-hand fighting skills developed by Yoshimitsu Minamoto. This system has been called Daito Ryu, also known as Daido Ryu, and it has always been considered the first form of Aikijujutsu.

The Okinawan warriors used this form of martial arts as the foundation for everything else. As other influences came to Okinawa, the warriors merged every aspect into their martial art. These included Shorinji Kempo of both Kenshojutsu, fist-palm art, and Goken, the five animal forms, as well as Taikyoku Ken (Tai Chi Chuan), Kei I (Hsing I), and Hakke Ken (Pa Kua). Another specific form is Hakutsuru Ken, white-crane form, which was influential in the development of several of the Shorin Ryu systems.

Although many Karate styles have a limited range of techniques because of an immersion in competition and the effects of modernization, some Kempo styles of Okinawa continue to teach the full range of skills, including throws, joint locks, chokes, strikes, punches, kicks, and weapons training.

Some Japanese styles of Kempo also teach the full range of skills, with some having accepted an influence from Okinawa to preserve a more complete set of self-defense skills. Other Japanese styles maintain a level of purity, punching and striking in the traditional Japanese manner, specifically without the five animal hand formations or the twisting punch so common to the Okinawan styles.

Regardless of whether Kempo is of Japanese style, Okinawan style, or Chinese methods, this form of martial art, especially when practiced as a system of self-defense, is complete and comprehensive. Most provide methods of Kihon, Kata, and Kumite. Some maintain other ancient practices most closely associated with combat effectiveness, specifically Renzoku Ken and Embu.

When James Masayoshi Mitose first brought Kempo to the continental United States, he emphasized Renzoku Ken training, which has become the mainstay of the Kempo styles in America. Embu, as practiced in the past in its original freestyle manner, is the specialized training of spontaneity so necessary to real combat and self-defense.

Go no Kempo

When Chinese martial arts came to Okinawa, they began to have an impact on the indigenous skills of the Okinawans. The Okinawans classified the Chugoku Kempo, Chinese martial arts, into two groups. The first was Go no Kempo, which literally translates as "the fist law of strength."

The Go no Kempo were those derived from Shaolin sources, which include not only the direct Shaolin temple martial arts but also variations. Some authorities believe that there were two specific Shaolin sources, whereas others think that there was only one.

What is commonly assumed is that most of the Shaolin influence came from the Fukien temple, the second Shaolin temple built. The environment in southern China, especially around water bodies, dictated that people use lower kicks for balance and emphasize hand techniques. This influence was especially evident in the martial arts of the Goju Ryu lineage.

Shorinji Kempo, as the Shaolin martial arts are known in Okinawa, were considered instrumental in the development of the Kempo and Karate styles that developed on the island. Because we know, however, that many Okinawan masters were great kickers, it is not possible for the influence to have been only from the southern Shaolin temple, which emphasized low kicks.

White Crane

Other southern styles also affected the martial arts in Okinawa, including certain southern white-crane styles that emphasized special Chin na, or Chinese grappling skills, and Hung Chia, the Hung family martial arts. These styles were also derived from the Shaolin tradition. Being taught in the south and, according to legend, being taught on boats, they also emphasize low, close-range kicks.

Finally, a white-crane style that some believe also influenced certain Okinawan styles is Wing Chun, the original style of Chugoku Kempo that Bruce Lee studied. Certain facets of Wing Chun are easily recognizable in some of the Okinawan Ryu. Some have suggested that Wing Chun was a style of Shaolin martial arts that ended up being taught to secular people during the Ching Dynasty. Therefore, it is possible that this was one of the low-kicking, southern Shaolin styles that influenced Okinawan Ryu.

At some point, however, northern Shaolin Chuanfa must have come to Okinawa because the high kicks were important to some of the styles of Kempo Karate. Several famous Okinawan kickers used high kicks and flying kicks. The northern Shorinji Kempo must have influenced these kicks because they would not have been part of either the southern styles or Japanese martial arts.

Some white-crane styles, particularly those associated with the north, also would have been high-kicking styles. We know that many Okinawan stylists consider white-crane a special form of Kempo and that in some of these styles the white-crane form, Hakutsuru Kata, has high kicks. This would presuppose a northern origin.

Go no Kempo styles were normally associated with the Shaolin temple and thus were Buddhist in origin. These styles emphasized physical fitness, technical proficiency, and deep natural breathing. This accent on the physical has led these martial arts to be referred to as the external styles, meaning that they emphasize the development of the body. Most of the Shorin Ryu styles are based on the Go no Kempo martial arts that entered Okinawa from China.

Ju no Kempo

Two explanations are offered for Ju no Kempo. The first is that the phrase refers to the Taoist martial arts that came to Okinawa from China. The second explanation is based on the meaning of Ju no Kempo, "the fist law of gentleness/yielding." Viewed this way, it could be inferred that the phrase refers to the Japanese Jujutsu influence on Okinawan martial arts.

Let us first deal with the Chinese explanation. We do not know when the Taoist martial arts entered Okinawa, but certain characteristics of the Okinawan styles clearly reflect their influence. Although certain movements, combinations, and applications of Karate skills can be interpreted in relation to the three internal arts, a definitive examination is nearly impossible for two reasons.

First, Buddhist and Taoist martial arts use some of the same movements. Looking only at exterior form is useless in determining the art of origin. It is impossible to distinguish a vertical fist punch of a Shaolin style from one of a Taoist style. A crescent kick has the same look whether performed by a Buddhist or a Taoist, especially when executed in actual fighting.

What makes a movement specifically Buddhist or Taoist is the philosophy behind it, the breathing style, and the way the person moves, either with or without tension. When the Okinawans learned movements from the Chinese sources, they changed them to fit their own ways of combat. In many cases they modified the methods or blended the two methods to achieve a synthesis that would better fit their physiology and psychology.

Yet we know specifically that two Ryu in Okinawa claim to have influence from the three Chinese Taoist martial arts. Before we deal with those Ryu, it might be pertinent to name and explain the three Taoist martial arts. These are sometimes referred to as internal style, meaning that they emphasize Ki (known in Chinese as Chi).

The oldest Taoist martial art is Tai Chi Chuan, which translates as the "grand ultimate fist." The reference is not to Tai Chi Chuan as the grand, ultimate martial art but to its reliance on the grand ultimate, which is the supreme principle of Taoism. In essence, it is the same concept as that of Shinken, the idea that the martial art comes from a divine source.

It is believed that Taoist monks saw the Buddhist monks maintaining good health and well-being through their martial art. Although they had excellent forms of exercise based on animal movements, the Taoist monks had not turned the exercises into combat methods. According to legend, one Taoist monk learned the Shaolin Chuanfa and applied Taoist principles to the forms, creating the Tai Chi Chuan. Like Shaolin, original Tai Chi did not have a set pattern. Instead it had a set of movements that could be combined in many ways in spontaneous motions. The main philosophical concept of Tai Chi is the balance and shifting of the Yin and the Yang.

According to certain sources, some people who practiced Tai Chi Chuan favored particular movements over others. One group favored the circular techniques and emphasized the concept of grappling. They developed a form of martial art based on the eight trigrams of the Taoist philosophy and created Pa Kua, which literally is "eight trigrams."

The other group preferred the more direct actions and created the art of Hsing I, "form of the will," which philosophically is based on the five elements. The group expanded the movements into a set called by the names of the 12 zodiac animals.

As fate would have it, at some point in history all three arts were drawn back together in another martial art, called I Chuan, or "will fist." Thus the Taoist martial arts went full circle, beginning with Tai Chi, breaking into three pieces, and reuniting in I Chuan.

According to some Okinawan historians, the Bushi of Okinawa adopted the three arts into the practice of their Bushi Te when the art entered the island, which was probably in the 19th century. It is believed that the Chin na, grappling skills of Tai Chi Chuan, and Pa Kua, in particular, affected the development of restraints and throws in the warrior martial art.

We know that Goju Ryu founder Chojun Miyagi traveled to China and studied an art called I Chuan. Some believe it was simply Hsing I called by another name, whereas others believe it was the triune Taoist martial art. Probably the latter is true because certain grappling skills preserved in Goju Ryu appear to be derived from Tai Chi or Pa Kua sources.

Thus it is possible that the three Taoist martial arts are being referred to by the term Ju no Kempo. But we should also look at the possibility that the Ju is derived from the Japanese Jujutsu influence.

The term Jujutsu was not used generically in Japan for empty-hand fighting until the 17th century, but certain Ryu used the term or the related pronunciation, Yawara, which is the common pronunciation for the Kanji, or character, Ju. We know that Tametomo Minamoto came to Okinawa in the 12th century, bringing with him the family Bujutsu, which included empty-hand fighting. Later, after the Minamoto defeated the Taira in Japan, some of the Taira fled to Okinawa, so that influence would have reached the island as well.

Muneomi Sawayama (1904–1993)

Muneomi Sawayama, a student of many of the martial arts of Japan, enjoyed the knowledge of Judo and Jujutsu of many Ryu. When Kenwa Mabuni of Okinawa came to Japan to teach, Sawayama saw the excitement of the new form of combat, which was at that time called Kempo Karate.

Sawayama, wishing to maintain his Japanese martial-arts skills, decided to merge his skills into the Kempo Karate curriculum he was learning under Mabuni. Sawayama created what he called "Nippon Kempo," a form of training that uses the throws of Judo, the joint locks of Jujutsu, and the striking skills of Karate. Nippon Kempo teaches very practical throws that, unlike Judo throws, don't require gripping the opponent's clothing. Some throws work by capturing the head, and there is also a throat throw. Nippon Kempo practitioners garb themselves in Kendo (swordsmanship) armor and fight in Kempo gloves, the kind made famous by Bruce Lee in the opening scenes of *Enter the Dragon*.

In 1609, the Satsuma first took over Okinawa through superior numbers and strategy. The Satsuma used a guerrilla force to capture the king while the Okinawan warriors were fighting the main body on the beach. The Japanese began to believe that the Okinawans were simple country bumpkins, unsophisticated and unknowledgeable.

Some of the Japanese Samurai eventually became close to the Okinawan royalty, to the point where they accepted some of the Samurai as students. History records that at least two of the great Okinawan martial-arts masters, Sokon Matsumura and Yasutsune Azato, held teaching certificates in the Jigen Ryu Bujutsu system of the Satsuma.

Some believe that the term Ju no Kempo was coined for all Japanese empty-hand fighting styles that came to Okinawa and influenced the maturing empty-hand systems. It is known that some martial artists actually used the term Jute, or "gentle hand," for their grappling art.

More than likely Ju no Kempo was used in reference to both aspects. Because the Taoist martial arts, especially Tai Chi and Pa Kua, emphasize Chin na, or grappling, as do the empty-hand systems of Japan, it is probable that the two sets of skills blended together and were basically combined into the one category of Ju no Kempo.

Kempo Karate

This phrase is well known in the United States today. We can trace the phrase back to Japan at the time when the Okinawan arts were first being taught before the development of the Okinawan Ryu, which occurred in the 1930s.

Several Okinawan instructors who taught in Japan wrote books in which they used the term Kempo Karate. They used both words because the Japanese would not have understood what Karate was. Karate was a common term on Okinawa but had never been seen outside the island. A Japanese person would see the word and not realize it applied to the martial arts. But

Japan had forms of Kempo going back at least to the 12th century when the monks in temples used the term for their warrior monk art. Some believe that Japanese forms of Kempo might be even older than that.

Thus when the Okinawan masters wrote books dealing with their form of combat, they used the term Kempo Karate to help people perusing titles in bookstores understand that the subject matter was martial arts.

We know that during this time, the great Okinawan masters—Gichin Funakoshi, Choki Motobu, and Kenwa Mabuni—all used the term Kempo Karate in their books. As time passed and the word Karate became the accepted term for Okinawan empty-hand fighting, many Japanese and Okinawan instructors dropped the word Kempo from the title.

But some masters, Choki Motobu in particular, felt that the complete term Kempo Karate was more descriptive of what he was teaching. Kempo, meaning "fist law," and Karate, meaning "empty hand," helped a prospective student understand that both the fist and the hand were effective weapons. The complete term thus helped a person appreciate the full range of weapons.

A second reason for using the full term Kempo Karate is that it encompasses a philosophical meaning. Kempo can have the expanded meaning of Ken, or "fist," alluding to the fact that as fingers join to form a fist, so must the nature of human join mind, body, and spirit to form a unified person. Ho, or "law," refers to the natural law of the universe (God). Thus the philosophical meaning of Kempo suggests a unified person following the natural law of the universe. This idea was regarded as the esoteric key to fighting skills. Everything that a Kempoka does should be natural. By following natural law, the martial artist can maximize his or her ability, move smoothly, and strike powerfully.

After 1903, Karate began to be written with the Kanji that meant "empty hand." Before this, it had been written with the characters that meant "Tang hand," referring to the Chinese Tang dynasty, when the martial arts were supposed to have reached their zenith. In 1936, a board of Okinawan masters voted that the characters meaning "empty hand" best described Okinawan martial arts.

Many have thought that the masters chose this meaning because Karate was a weaponless form of fighting. But this observation is incorrect. Okinawan martial arts employ many weapons, and the masters chose the term because of its philosophical meaning. Kara, or "empty," alludes to the emptiness of the Void, that which is beyond the phenomenal world. Thus Kara has the same connotation as "losing oneself in God" has to the Western world. Te, as stated earlier, can be used to mean "hand," "skill," or "person." Thus Karate is the skill of finding the Void. It may also refer to a person who has found the Void.

Therefore, Kempo Karate can mean simply the "fist law, empty-hand form of fighting" or esoterically "the unified person follows the natural law of the universe (God) and finds himself one with the Void (God)."

The term was first used in the United States when Hawaii was still a territory. Chojun Miyagi, an Okinawan master, was invited to the island in 1934 to teach martial arts for a year. A newspaper announcing his coming used the phrase Kempo Karate. This phrase stayed with the Hawaiian students. Years later it was revitalized and used by many people in reference to the martial arts that developed on the island. Eventually, Ed Parker, a student of William Chow, who trained under James Masayoshi Mitose, brought Kempo to the continental United States and taught it under the name Kempo Karate.

Today the Kempo lineage derived from Mitose is one of the largest groups in America. Although no unified Kempo body exists, many groups, most of which use the term Kempo Karate, evolved from this single lineage, a line that goes back to the great Okinawan master Choki Motobu, one of the teachers of James Masayoshi Mitose.

Nippon Kempo

In Japan, as the term Jujutsu came to be used generically for all empty-hand forms of fighting, the various terms originally used by the Ryu and in the temples began to fall into disuse. Among the terms originally used for empty-hand fighting in Japan are Kempo, Torite, Wajutsu, Taijutsu, Kogusoku, Kumi Uchi, Yawara, Gotenjutsu, and Oshikiuchi.

Use of the term Kempo was preserved in the temples but rarely used outside of them until modern times. Two main influences led to the revival of the term Kempo in modern Japan. The first, as earlier noted, was the potency of Kempo Karate of Okinawa. After seeing the effectiveness of the Okinawan martial art, several Japanese martial artists decided to create a Japanese variation while at the same time researching their roots and discovering more about Japanese forms of Kempo.

Some historians noted that such ancient systems of combat as Kito Ryu, Tenshin Shinyo Ryu, Araki Ryu, Ryoi Shinto Ryu, Fukuno Ryu, and others had a well-developed striking curriculum generally called Kempo. Some of these forms, particularly the Kito Ryu, Ryoi Shinto Ryu, and Fukuno Ryu, seemed to build almost exclusively on Kempo.

With this knowledge and influence from the Okinawan martial art, two Japanese Kempo organizations developed. One was simply called Nippon Kempo, and the other was termed Nippon Goshindo Kempo, with Goshindo meaning "the way of self-defense."

Both arts include a complete curriculum of techniques, including throwing, joint locking, striking, kicking, and so on. Nippon Kempo focuses on a type of full-contact sparring in which practitioners wear special gloves and Kendo-like armor. Zenryo Shimabuku and Shigeru Nakamura of the Okinawan Kempo Kai pioneered this form of training, and the Nippon Kempo practitioners adopted it.

The second influence on the resurgence of the term Kempo among Japanese martial artists was the development of Nippon Shorinji Kempo. As noted earlier, Michiomi Nakano trained in Shorinji Kempo during his days as a spy before and during World War II (also known as the Pacific War). Being named the successor, he returned to Japan after the war. He trained in a Daito Ryu

Aikijujutsu Dojo for a time before finally establishing his own school and creating the style of Nippon Shorinji Kempo.

In an interesting development, Chinese practitioners of the Shaolin Chuanfa charged Nakano with fraud because his Shorinji Kempo did not look like their Shaolin, lacking the five animal forms that modern Shaolin is famous for. They petitioned the government and demanded that Nakano change the name of his art.

After Nakano established his martial art and founded a new religion called Kongo Zen, students flocked to his temple school. He had literally hundreds of students practicing Nippon Shorinji Kempo. In Japan, Nakano's form of Kempo is regarded as one of the most effective of all fighting styles. This reputation has helped create an interest not only in his form of Kempo but in others as well.

Modern Kempo has its roots in China. From there it spread over the centuries to Japan, Korea, Okinawa, Hawaii, and the continental United States. As Kempo changed through varied cultures, combat applications, and modernization, several distinct forms of Kempo emerged.

Kempo Tradition

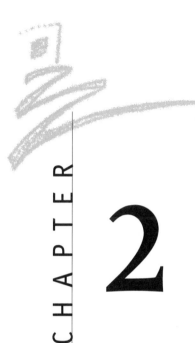

Kempo tradition is deep. Over the centuries, Kempoka developed five traditional training methods. All require practice at different levels and attention to safety.

TRADITIONAL TRAINING METHODS

Five traditional methods of Kempo training form the foundation of martial-arts practice. Some systems use other names, but here we use Kihon, Kumite, Renzoku Ken, Kata, and Embu. Kumite and Renzoku Ken are sometimes known as Waza, or techniques.

The foundation of everything in the martial arts are the concepts of Kihon and Kata. Kumite, Renzoku Ken, and Waza are methods of applying basic movements in self-defense with a partner.

Kihon: The Basics

Training in the martial arts begins with Kihon, which provides the foundation for proper development. Kihon plays the same role in martial arts that the alphabet does in language or numerals do in mathematics. Regardless of rank, the best Kempoka constantly work on their Kihon, striving to improve their fundamental movements.

Kihon teaches the basic movement and helps the Kempoka understand the principle behind the concept of motion. It is important that the practitioner focus on mastering the principle while developing physical control of the body. Kempo is as much an intellectual pursuit as it is a physical discipline. The higher the rank, the more intellectual the training. Nevertheless, one must not forget that a martial artist is first a physical person. Fitness is an essential aspect of being a true martial artist.

The Kihon in most Kempo styles consists primarily of movements that the beginner interprets as blocks, strikes, and kicks. As a beginner, the Kempoka starts with simple Kihon, using inner circular blocks, outer circular blocks, reverse punches, knife hands, elbow strikes, front kicks, roundhouse kicks, and side kicks. The person who advances to the senior ranks learns to lunge, spin, twist, leap, and slide using each of the basic movements and more advanced skills.

At each level, all the way up through the lower grades of black belt, Kempoka learn new, advanced Kihon that push them and challenge their physical and mental abilities. Yet even as a person progresses, he or she is expected to keep improving previous Kihon. In some styles, Yudansha, black-belt holders, are expected to take pretests before being considered for a subsequent rank. They must demonstrate all their old Kihon before being tested on their new skills.

Kumite: Sparring

After a person learns the Kihon for a particular rank, he or she must learn how to apply them in basic sparring, in what is called Kihon Kumite. In this method of training, a partner throws a certain attack to which the defender responds with the required technique. Some Kihon Kumite are simple, such as the outer circular block used to counter the attacking partner's roundhouse punch. Other Kihon Kumite are more complex, such as the reverse punch. Here the attacker launches a lunge punch, and the defender dodges to the front corner, cross blocks, and counters with a reverse punch.

The term Kumite is usually translated today as "sparring," but this meaning is misleading because it causes people to think that Kempo or Karate is nothing more than a method of boxing with kicks, a conception far from the truth.

Sparring is a word in English that intimates the idea of a controlled, yet freestyle, fight. We think of boxers practicing with a sparring partner, a person who takes hits and hits back, but not too hard. Still, most people consider sparring a fight with intensity ranging from light contact to full contact.

Kempo was not traditionally practiced this way in the Orient, particularly in the Okinawan method. Literally, Kumite means "unite with, cooperate with, or grapple with." Sparring connotes people striking at one another, whereas the implied meaning of Kumite is a coming together of two practitioners. Usually translated as "grappling hand," Kumite denotes two people practicing together.

By understanding that the term Kumi means "cooperate with" and that Te can mean not only "hand" but also "person" or "people," then we see that Kumite can actually mean "cooperate with person," with a training partner. This is the way it was used in Okinawa in years past to stand for martial-arts training. Kumite was a cooperative method between two Kempoka.

In original Kumite, two practitioners would take turns as attacker and defender. The defender would tell the attacker what kind of technique to strike with and then spontaneously defend against it. They would then switch roles. At times, the Kempoka would have a list of different attacks, performing them and developing defenses against each.

A defender usually made only one strike in return against an attack because the main principle of the Okinawan martial arts was Ikken Hissatsu—one strike, certain death. Although practitioners did not necessarily seek to kill, it was felt that if the technique was powerful and the hit focused over a vital point, death was a certainty. This is another reason that Okinawan martial artists did not believe in fighting.

Kumite in the old days were conducted in two other ways. One was for the attacker to launch an assault, which the defender blocked. Then the attacker would launch another blow. The defender would counter and perform a finishing blow. In many situations, a whole scenario was designed, so that a defender could learn how to counter a series of strikes. This type of Kumite might have been derived from the Embu, which came to Okinawa from Shaolin Chuanfa. The great Kempo Karate master Choki Motobu was particularly famous for this form of Kumite.

Kumite, in the practice of the original, combat-oriented Kempo, was never intended to be a match or fight between two martial artists. The Okinawans considered the art too dangerous for such a game of combat. Most of all, they realized that with the medicine of the time, injuries suffered in fights could lead to disability or death. Thus the Kumite of Kempo in the past was a cooperative way of training safely in the skills of self-defense.

Kyusho: Vital Points

Kihon Kumite helps people understand how to apply the basic movements in actual self-defense. The study of Kihon Kumite introduces students to Kyusho, the vital points. No strike is ever just launched in the general direction of the opponent. Instead, the practitioner aims specifically at a vital point on the body of the opponent—nerve centers, blood vessels, joint weaknesses, body cavities, and acupressure points.

Bunkai: Analysis

To aim a strike, one must use the advanced concept called Bunkai. Each move can have many interpretations; a practitioner can use a single move in different ways to strike various Kyusho. What is commonly thought of as a block may be used as a strike, and many strikes can be blocks. Kicks are normally strikes, but one can also use kicks to block certain attacks. Any weapon can strike many points on the body or an attacking limb, thus making hits and blocks much more effective.

Many people do not commonly practice the use of blocks, strikes, and kicks as throws, chokes, and joint locks. At black-belt grades, therefore, great emphasis is placed on Bunkai. The Okinawans developed this process of analysis to an exceptional level.

Renzoku Ken: Techniques

Another type of Kumite was known as Renzoku Ken. In Renzoku Ken, an attacker would launch an assault that the defender assumed could not be handled by one blow. Although they trained to stop an attacker with one punch, the Okinawans were realists and knew that this would not always be possible. Thus they trained to put combinations together fluidly.

These combinations could be made up of hand strikes or kicks and strikes. At advanced levels, the combinations could contain throws and joint locks, and possibly even chokes and other skills. Kempoka developed the most advanced skills in Renzoku Ken. When Kempo came to the United States, this was the most exciting and appealing facet of the art to those who saw it performed.

Renzoku Ken is a serious method of training that requires the practitioner to combine all skills logically. Renzoku Ken is what most people think of as Kempo. From the Okinawan perspective, each movement should be capable of putting a person down. This is referred to as Ikken, or "one fist." In the ancient times this was called Ikken Hissatsu, literally "one fist, certain death."

But the Okinawans understood that if the attacker was strong enough, if the defender missed the vital point that he or she was aiming for, or if other factors intervened, then one strike might not stop an opponent. Thus they trained to perform a continuous flow of strikes.

Renzoku Ken is one of the main principles of all forms of Kempo in America, although as stated earlier it is known by many names and sometimes referred to simply as techniques. In the development of Renzoku Ken, no prearranged sets should be present, according to the teachings of James Masayoshi Mitose. When he published his classic book *What is Self Defense? Kempo JiuJitsu* in 1953, Mitose originally wanted only a philosophy book. Instead, pictures illustrated the edition. He performed freestyle skills for the book, but readers have since believed that what he showed were prearranged techniques of his form of Kempo. Thus as masters established their own systems, they created set patterns, not realizing that they were breaking one of the main principles of original Kempo training—Mukei, or "no set form."

In some styles, students are expected to learn how to create their own combinations spontaneously from the Kihon and Kihon Kumite that they learn from their instructors. In some systems, students must have the ability to create Renzoku Ken spontaneously to progress through the black-belt levels.

Symmetry

In the development of Renzoku Ken, a person must develop a symmetry of movement, a constant flow of motion that allows each move to blend smoothly into the next, without interruption. When the student can do this, the opponent has no time or opportunity to recover and mount a defense.

Elvis Presley (1935–1977)

Considered by many the greatest entertainer who ever lived, Presley thrilled the world with his beautiful singing and light-hearted movies. His popularity skyrocketed in the 1970s with his return to live performances. It was with the help of karate that "the King" was able to create his own harmony and balance his life and his fame. Presley began his training in the martial arts during his service in the military, learning Judo, Jujutsu, and Karate. He earned his Shodan under Hank Slemansky in 1960 at Memphis, Tennessee.

In Hollywood, later that year, he met Ed Parker and began working with him. Over the years, Presley also trained with Bill "Superfoot" Wallace and Kang Rhee. Most of his best friends and bodyguards were also practitioners of the martial arts and served as training partners during his time away from movie shoots and recording sessions.

Many have said that Elvis cherished Karate second only to his music. He once expressed a desire to teach Karate, although his fame prohibited such a public enterprise. He did run a Karate school in conjunction with Red West and Bill "Superfoot" Wallace. His Tennessee Karate Institute taught a combination of Kempo and Karate.

Those who trained with and saw Elvis perform Kempo and Karate had no doubt about his knowledge and ability. He performed martial arts in many of his films during a time when people knew little about them. He sponsored many martial artists and martial-arts activities. During his life, Elvis did a great deal to popularize the martial arts. At his death, he was an eighth-degree black belt under the auspices of Ed Parker.

Connectedness

Renzoku Ken is also a time of intense Bunkai training that teaches the advanced student how to see the connectedness of movement. This also results from Kata training, in which the student spontaneously combines moves that he or she can then try in Renzoku Ken practice.

Practical Training

During Renzoku Ken practice, the student will see how distance and timing can convert a block, strike, or kick into a throw or joint lock. This practical training involving another person is what allows the Kempoka to keep his or her skills grounded in reality. The student must spend time with a partner to ensure that the movements work as the practitioner has analyzed they will.

Kata: Form

At all levels of rank, the most important method of practice is Kata, which translates as "form," "pattern," or "style." There are two types of Kata.

Freestyle

The most ancient form is freestyle, which has no set pattern to the movements. Forms of freestyle Kata were always methods of combat training that quickly prepared people for the realism of fighting. Freestyle Kata has roots as far back as China, and it was used in both Japan and Okinawa during the warring eras.

Prearranged Form

The second type of Kata, the prearranged form, is more common. These forms are generally preset movements, practiced the same way in each performance.

Prearranged Kata could be taught to a person without teaching him or her how to fight, unless they were also taught Bunkai. The Kempo teachers of Okinawa could thus instruct their students without worrying about their young charges misusing the art. Prearranged Kata also provide an easy way to grade the students because if they could demonstrate the prearranged movements of their Kata, they would pass.

The original idea of the Okinawans was to develop in their young students a high level of physical fitness during training. When they were older, they could enter a Dojo, a martial-arts school. Under a Kempo Karate master, they would learn the Bunkai of the movements of their prearranged Kata. When they were ready, the master would teach them the advanced freestyle Kata.

Unfortunately, the Japanese who picked up Karate focused on the prearranged sets and created the sport form of Karate, fixing it into a mold that has almost caused the extinction of the original Kempo of Okinawa. Today, many styles of Kempo include only prearranged Kata in their curriculums. Most of the Japanese and Okinawan styles use the same Kata as most Shorin Ryu Karate systems. Some forms of Chinese-based Kempo use the prearranged sets of various styles of Shaolin.

Masters of contemporary Kempo have developed many modern forms. Some are designed for competition, with little combat realism in their movements. Others are more realistically designed for self-defense. Many of the movements of Kempo are based on the five animal techniques of the original Goken Shorinji Kempo from China. Taught properly, these movements offer excellent self-defense skills.

Beginners learn basic Kata, whether of the Jiyu or Yakusoku type. As the person advances, the Kata become more complex, with greater levels of sophistication and complexity. As with the Kihon, however, students are expected to maintain command of their old Kata. Those worthy of their Kempo ranks do not permit any of their old skills to deteriorate.

Embu: Partners

An aspect of Kempo that did not make the transition to the United States until the early 1980s is Embu, one of the most creative and educational forms of training. The difference between sparring and Embu is that in the latter form of practice the two Kempoka view each other as partners, working in harmony so that both improve. In competition, one fighter attempts to defeat the other. This objective is at odds with the original principle of the martial arts, which, as noted earlier, is to stop violence. All too often competition encourages an aggressive attitude that can promote conflict in daily life. According to Michiomi Nakano (So Doshin), the great founder of Nippon Shorinji Kempo, Embu was a method of practice used at the original Shaolin temple in China. This method allowed the Buddhist monks to practice their martial art with a partner without brutality or competition.

Embu did not make an easy transition to the United States because by the time Kempo made it to the continent, the Japanese had developed sport Karate, which appealed to the competitive nature of the Western world. Thus, besides Kihon Kumite, the American martial artist primarily practiced Jiyu Kumite, or free sparring, which was developed by the Japanese.

Embu as a discipline is found in Nippon Shorinji Kempo and Kiyojute Ryu Kempo Bugei, as well as in many styles of Aikido and Kobujutsu. The modern Kempo practitioner would find it advantageous to learn this special form of training.

Peaceful Mind

In Embu, Kempoka learn how to apply their techniques in a constant exchange of movements while maintaining a mind of peace and harmony. The Kempoka is never to become angry or express hatred toward an opponent. Instead, he or she should defend with a passive mind that desires no harm toward anyone.

Attack and Counterattack

Embu starts with one practitioner initiating an attack. The other person dodges or blocks and then performs a counterattack, which too is countered. The result is a constant exchange of skill. To eliminate chance of injury, practitioners

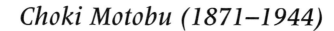

Choki Motobu (1871–1944)

Choki Motobu, the great Kempo Karate master from Okinawa, was once visiting Japan when a European heavyweight boxer was giving demonstration bouts. The boxer was accepting all challengers and beating them easily. Choki's Japanese friend asked if Choki thought any martial artists on Okinawa could beat the boxer. Motobu replied "five or six." Incredulous, his friend asked how the tiny island of Okinawa could have that many good martial artists, when all the Japanese fighters were losing to the boxer.

Choki was somewhat offended that his Japanese friend didn't believe him, so when the boxer called out for another challenger, Choki stood up and accepted. Choki was 56 years old at the time and had never seen western boxing before. He climbed into the ring and dodged the boxer for a while. He then hit the boxer so hard that he went down and had to be carried out of the ring.

This event made Choki Motobu instantly famous. The Japanese regarded him as the greatest fighter in the world, and he immediately had many Japanese martial artists seeking him out for lessons. Practitioners of other martial arts came to him to add the Kempo Karate of Okinawa to their Bujutsu curriculum.

Choki's fame made him truly feel like the greatest in the world. He went back home to Okinawa, wanting his people to know how successful and famous he had become. He visited his older brother, Choyu, and told him the whole story. Choyu congratulated Choki, sharing in his joy. With a smile, Choki then challenged his brother to a match.

Back in those days there was no such thing as a sparring match as we think of today. Rather, a match involved a test of strength, through a type of wrestling called *tegumi* (hand matching) or *teawase* (hand facing). Choki, the larger of the two brothers, felt invincible. The match began as the two brothers faced each other and bowed. Choki used his famed footwork to bring him into contact with his brother, where he hoped his superior strength and great skill would allow him to overpower his brother, but each time he came into range, he was hurled to the ground. Those who witnessed the battle said it seemed as if Choyu was toying with his brother, throwing him at will and keeping him helpless. This is the great power of the Torite.

pull strikes one inch from contact. Because there is no contact, practitioners can target vital points, making this a highly effective method of self-defense training. Although strikes are the primary techniques of interchange, Kempoka can also use throws and joint locks in the exercise. In some styles, the practitioner combines a throw or joint lock with a finishing movement, either a clearing movement or strike, to end the Embu.

Thus, to learn Kempo correctly, students must follow the comprehensive program that has been passed down through the generations of Kempo masters, starting with Bodhidharma and going through to James Masayoshi Mitose, who brought it to the United States and passed it on to his students. They, in turn, shared it with the rest of the country and the world.

Kempo training begins with Kihon, progresses to Kihon Kumite, and advances to Kata. Kihon Kumite and Embu are two important forms of training because the student practices them with a partner. Students can thus see the development of their techniques in actual application against a person.

Kempo has always been a comprehensive martial art that uses a logical progression of training to develop a high level of skill and ability in its practitioners. Although terms may differ according to primary heritage (Chinese, Japanese, or Okinawan), the training methods are the same—Kihon, Kihon Kumite, Kata, Renzoku Ken, and Embu.

THE THREE FACES OF KEMPO

Many people want to know the secret of martial-arts training, especially those who train in Kempo. The secret is simple—one must practice. In a most mundane interpretation, the three faces of Kempo—Renshu, Keiko, and Shugyo—mean practice, "practice, practice."

Each form of Kempo has a foundation, be it either Chinese, Japanese, Okinawan, or even Korean. When one begins to study a form of Kempo, it is important to ask questions and learn about its lineage. Because all the branches of Kempo are similar, it is obvious that they have a common root. In ancient times that would have been the Shaolin temple. In modern times, it is the Mitose lineage, which goes back to Okinawa and the great masters of Kempo Karate.

One must understand that every martial-arts term in the Japanese language possesses a profound interpretation as well as a mundane one. In ancient times, the masters kept their lesser students and untrustworthy disciples from achieving complete knowledge by withholding the esoteric understanding of the terms. Without that information, a student's training was not complete.

Amazingly, most of the esoteric teachings were based on spiritual matters, for the spirit lies at the heart of true progress and the potential for greatness. Without these spiritual instructions, a student could at best become only a proficient athlete. It was the esoteric meaning of the martial-arts terms that allowed the martial artist to achieve mastery.

Each of these three words—Renshu, Keiko, and Shugyo—is composed of two Kanji. By understanding what the root characters mean, we can have a full understanding of real Kempo training.

Renshu: Practice

The first word, Renshu, is made up of Ren, meaning "to polish," and Shu, meaning "take lessons." Thus the first admonition from the term Renshu is to take lessons and polish the skills. If the student refuses to practice, lessons taught by even the finest teacher go unlearned. All the greatest masters, from Mitose, Ueshiba, and Kano to Funakoshi, Motobu, and Kyan, had mediocre students. Each of them had many outstanding students as well, who went on to become masters in their own right. Thus, although top students proved their methods of teaching worthy, even the masters had students who would not work hard and practice what they had been taught.

Renshu lets us know how important it is to have a good teacher, yet it also tells us that we must polish what we have been taught. Stories in the history of the martial arts recount that mediocre teachers with little knowledge have students who work so hard on everything they are taught that one day they become great masters, far outstripping their teachers. Although such an occurrence is rare, it has happened occasionally because of the Renshu, the practicing of the material given.

Renshu also explains how some students who were denied entry to a school, such as the great Tai Chi master Yang and Kempo Karate great Choki Motobu, could watch their teachers train and then secretly practice what they saw until their skills were so great that the teachers had to accept them as their pupils.

The need to polish one's skills is the most important lesson a beginner in the martial arts can learn. Nothing in this world, no secret knowledge, no special instruction, can take the place of old-fashioned practice.

Keiko: Practice

For the intermediate student of Kempo, practice is just as important, but it now takes on a new idea, that of Keiko. Kei means "think, consider," and Ko means "old." Thus the admonition from Keiko is simply "think of the old." This is the idea behind Bunkai, which we will deal with more fully later, but in simple terms it is looking at what you already know as if you are seeing it for the first time.

For example, Keiko means to take something like a reverse punch and look at it as if you were learning for the first time, although you have been training for 20 years. This may sound ridiculous, but it allows the Kempoka to see aspects of the technique that he or she may have forgotten or never understood. Again using the idea of the reverse punch, a beginner learned how to punch straight ahead with the reverse punch to strike someone in front of him or her. An intermediate student might consider the same technique and begin thinking about all the angles with which he or she might use it. The student may suddenly discover cross punches, side punches, descending punches, and more. Even an advanced practitioner with 15 or 20 years of training might start to find in the simple reverse punch such grappling skills as reverse wristlocks, wrist rotations, arm stretches, entering throws, and more.

No matter what level a person reaches in the martial arts, he or she must keep practicing. In fact, the longer a person has been in the martial arts, the greater the need for Keiko because he or she has so much more to think about. True Kempo masters have incredibly intricate and sophisticated skills only because they have been contemplating for 20 or 30 years the techniques they learned in the first 5 years of training.

Some would have you believe that the training concerns only the mental aspects. But it also involves dedicated physical training, going through the moves of the old techniques to glean a greater understanding of their meanings. One cannot achieve this by sitting around thinking of the skills. It is necessary to be up and moving, meditating on the movements.

At this level, the movements are themselves a great form of moving meditation that helps the student grow spiritually. At the same time, the student deepens his or her knowledge and ability in the physical art of Kempo.

Shugyo: Practice

This leads to the highest level of practice, known by the term Shugyo. This term has a rich and varied history that begins outside martial-arts training. Originally, it was used for the practice of religious austerities, such as forms of discipline designed to increase spiritual growth. Shugyo combined with Sha, meaning "person," is Shugyosha, which generally refers to a practitioner of Buddhist austerities.

Because many martial arts began in Buddhist temples and because Kempo was considered a form of hard work, it too became regarded as a method of austerities. As the martial art left the temple and members of the laity began to practice it, the term went with it too. Thus anyone who trained hard in any martial art was encouraged to Shugyo.

Let us look again at the deeper meaning of this word. Shu, written with a different Kanji than in Renshu, means to "govern oneself, conduct oneself well, study, cultivate, or master." Gyo by itself can literally mean "religious austerities," but it can also have the connotation of "exercise control" or "act."

Thus Shugyo can mean to "exercise control to conduct oneself well," or "through religious austerities one should govern oneself," or "act with cultivation." All carry with them the idea of study and the goal of achieving mastery.

In many martial-arts schools, the idea of Shugyo can be summed up in English as "work hard." Although this carries an admirable meaning, one must consider the idea of religious austerities and the goal of masterly self-conduct.

In an age when too many people comport themselves poorly and when many martial artists exhibit poor sporting behavior and irascible conduct during competitions, a return to the idea of Shugyo would be beneficial. Shugyo gives a connotation of spiritual development, which in the Orient has always meant an evolution of moral conduct.

Shugyo as a form of religious austerities does not have the connotation of dogma or doctrine. Instead, it points to a whole-hearted dedication to training with the body, mind, and spirit. It is a concept of total involvement with the goal of mastering oneself and achieving self-control.

In essence, the words Renshu, Keiko, and Shugyo are simple to translate—practice, practice, practice. But true Kempoka and all martial artists must know their esoteric meanings: Renshu, "take lessons and polish your skills"; Keiko, "think of the old"; and Shugyo, "through religious austerities one should govern oneself."

SAFE PRACTICE AND REAL COMBAT

Sun Dome, Hyomen Dome, Hyomen Hakai, and Naibu Hakai are the most important words in the practice of Kempo. The first two are about safe practice, and the last two are about life and death in combat. One must learn these concepts well to keep training partners safe and have the real power necessary to defend oneself.

Safety

When training with a partner in the forms of Kihon Kumite, Renzoku Ken, and Embu, it is important that one keeps skills in control so that no one is hurt. Keep in mind that each punch, strike, or kick in Kempo has the potential to do serious damage if it lands against a vital point of another person. This means that careless techniques are a danger in training.

Sun Dome: One Inch From Contact

The Okinawans developed the idea of Sun Dome, stopping a technique one inch from contact to eliminate the danger that a partner would be injured. In Kihon Kumite and Renzoku Ken, the partner, after launching an attack, remains still. The defender can then perform the single response, as in Kihon Kumite, or the multiple response, as in Renzoku Ken, without having to worry that the partner will accidentally move into a technique. Some consider this unrealistic, but weighed against ensuring the safety of one's training partner, it is understandable.

In Embu, as the partners move back and forth in the give-and-take method of training, each stops moving during the countermove of the partner to ensure safety. When the training partner pulls the technique, Sun Dome, and the target person is stationary, training in the techniques is perfectly safe.

Beginners should move slowly during the training so that they can judge distance accurately and stop one inch short of the target. Advanced black belts can move with full speed and power because they have the control to stop their blows one inch from contact. For the safety of one's partner, the student must never move faster than he or she can stop.

Hyomen Dome: Surface Stopping

Some Chinese and Japanese Kempo stylists use another method of safety training that we can refer to as Hyomen Dome, which means "surface stopping." Here the technique is allowed to touch the partner's body, but the force literally dissipates at the surface of the person's body.

Although Hyomen Dome is a viable way for advanced practitioners to train, it is dangerous for beginners. The practitioner must train for many years to achieve control sufficient to ensure that no force damages the partner's body. Even with advanced practitioners, accidents have occurred, especially when moving at full or normal speed. Therefore, it is my opinion that those training with partners should use Sun Dome only. Hyomen Dome is safe only when used at slow speeds.

Combat

Knowing that safe practice is dependent on Dome, or "stopping," within one inch or at the surface of the body, many people wonder how the martial arts work in actual self-defense. We find the answers in the ideas of Hyomen Hakai, Naibu Hakai, and Kime.

Let us start with Kime, which literally means "decisiveness" but refers to focus. The idea is that when a Kempoka decides where to put a technique, nothing stops him or her from going to that point. One develops this first with the eyes, looking where the punch, strike, or kick is supposed to go and then taking it there. Later, at advanced levels, it is possible to "see" the target with the mind's eye and move accordingly.

Once the Kempoka masters the idea of Kime, he or she applies it in Kihon Kumite, Renzoku Ken, and Embu by focusing one inch from the partner. Finally, the practitioner should use visualization to achieve both Hyomen Hakai and Naibu Hakai.

Hyomen Hakai: Bodily Damage

First, Hyomen Hakai means "surface destruction," destroying exterior parts of a person's body. The most easily understood example of Hyomen Hakai is damaging the nose. The nose protrudes on the face and can be smashed, broken, or ripped in actual self-defense. The main aspect of Hyomen Hakai is that although the damage can be extensive, painful, and debilitating, it is generally not life threatening.

Surface destruction can cause everything from bruising, stunning, and light bleeding, to body parts such as the nose and ears, being ripped off. Many Hyomen Hakai strikes cause continuous pain or damage them so that a limb becomes nearly useless. A strong surface strike can cause temporary paralysis to certain muscle groups, such as the diaphragm. When the diaphragm is stunned with a surface blow, the person receiving it cannot breathe. Because the blow is on the surface, however, the effect is only temporary.

Thus Hyomen Hakai is the appropriate response by a Kempoka who believes that he or she is more skillful than an attacker and is not worried about offering a defense in a confrontation. Hyomen Hakai is especially useful in one-on-one situations. But in multiple-attacker situations, or when facing a person of far superior size, or when meeting an obviously experienced opponent, then one should use the deadliest of striking concepts, Naibu Hakai.

Naibu Hakai: The Deadliest Concept

It has been said that this concept originally entered Okinawa from China, where it was developed by the Shaolin monks. It is believed, however, that the Okinawans developed the concept to its highest level. Various explanations are offered about how Naibu Hakai works, some very esoteric, others more fantasy than fact, but some are simple to understand.

Some claim that Naibu Hakai is the fact behind the legend of the Dim Mak, the so-called delayed death touch. In Japanese, Dim Mak is pronounced Ten Myaku and means "point on a blood vessel." Delayed death touch is a fabrication and misrepresentation of an intelligent, though brutal, technique.

First, we hear of the fanciful concept of shutting down, or turning on, the flow of energy through the body. Although an energy force definitely exists within the human body, it is of a spiritual nature and is usually referred to as Ki. The existence of a physical ability that can affect this spiritual energy is highly suspect.

The second unlikely theory is that blows performed on a person set up a vibration that travels through the person's body, doing damage as it goes. Neither of these concepts explains why Dim Mak sometimes works and sometimes does not. Likewise, neither theory explains the physical experience of the person who has been hit. Finally, for the process to work, both concepts demand an extremely high level of skill, experience, and personal knowledge about the victim. For example, with the idea of Dim Mak one must know the birthday and physical rhythms of the assailant to make an effective strike. A person would be unlikely to know such information about a spontaneous attacker, especially a stranger, thus making it impractical for self-defense.

Some will say that the delayed death touch will be effective only after 30 years of practice. So much for immediate self-defense. What is the secret of Okinawan training that allows a young person to have so much power and ability? The answer is focus of the mind and its application in the manner of Naibu Hakai. We have already talked about the focus of the mind, about Kime. The way one applies it is Naibu Hakai.

Naibu means "inner," and Hakai, as noted earlier, is "destruction." Naibu Hakai refers to using focus to project the power of the given strike in a compression of the body. The result is internal damage, usually from the collapse of blood vessels, pressure around nerves, and rupture of internal organs.

In ancient times, the Okinawans talked about Ikken Hissatsu—one hit, certain death—from their understanding of Ten Myaku and Naibu Hakai. It is possible to hit with such penetration that anything within the strike area is so severely damaged that the person will have a debilitating injury that could end in death.

Those who have been hit with a Naibu Hakai strike have told about feeling the hit at the point of contact but feeling the power on the other side of the body. This has been called a Ki Shindo, or energy pulse, a vibration that carries through the whole body from the force of the blow. This logical concept can be understood scientifically.

This may have been the origin of the concept of the vibrating palm. The hit causes the damage, but with internal bleeding and interior damage, death comes later, hence the idea of a delayed death.

Naibu Hakai is a matter of learning how to hit with penetration of one to two inches on the human body. Strikes can be simulated with a heavy bag, punching mitts, or Makiwari "striking post." The Kempoka must also learn where to hit by understanding the vital points of the human body. Such knowledge will help provide the greatest effectiveness in self-defense.

Kihon, Kumite, Kata, Renzoku Ken, and Embu are the five basic traditional training methods employed in Kempo. These methods are practiced at three levels—Renshu, Keiko, and Shugyo. Using these methods ensures safe practice and develops the ability to engage in real combat.

Kempo as a martial art and a lifestyle embodies many different techniques and training methods. Finding a balance between practicing safety and being able to defend oneself against an enemy requires patience, skill, and respect for one's partner, environment, ancestry, and ability.

Tachi:
The Stances

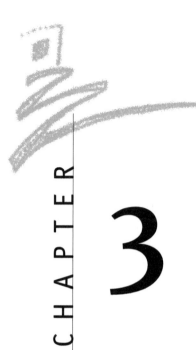

CHAPTER

3

Kempo, like most martial arts, has a foundation in stances. All techniques begin with proper footwork. Yet one does not stand still in self-defense. Instead, he or she moves constantly. Thus stance, known in the Japanese language as Tachi, is not a static concept, but a fluid one.

A secondary aspect of Tachi is Kamae, which can be translated as "posture" and deals with the whole body. In contrast, Tachi deals primarily with foot placement and leg position. Some styles use both terms; others do not. Moreover, some styles use Tachi and Kamae interchangeably, both referring to the position of the entire body.

A Kempoka's center, located two inches below the navel, is referred to as the Itten, or "one point." It is the center of the Hara, or abdominal area, which in the Orient is considered the seat of the soul. All movement in the martial arts begins in this center. It is essential that Kempoka keep themselves centered so they will be balanced and able to draw on their full strength. When a person's center is broken, he or she becomes weak and is easily thrown. The goal of all stance training is to keep one's center.

PRIMARY STANCES

In general, Kempo practitioners assume three stances. All others flow from these in movement and combat. The three primary stances are the natural stance, the defense stance, and the horse stance.

Natural Stance

Defense Stance

Horse Stance

Shizen Dachi: Natural Stance

The natural stance can be called Shizen Dachi. The feet are shoulder-width apart, and the weight is evenly distributed between them. This is the normal stance a person uses when waiting in a line, standing at ease, or just standing up.

This is an essential stance because we are in this position most of the time in life. To develop mastery, a person should learn how to move quickly and spontaneously from the natural stance. The Kempoka should devote enough time to working in Shizen Dachi so that he or she can move efficiently from this normal posture into any Kempo skill, whether it be throwing, locking, or striking.

Forewarned is forearmed, however, and the person who perceives danger can assume a safer position. Regarded as a variation of Shizen Dachi in the Japanese Kempo styles, this position has either the left foot forward, Hidari Shizen Dachi, or the right foot forward, Migi Shizen Dachi. The foot position is also known as Renoji Dachi in the Okinawan styles because the back foot is at a 45-degree angle to the front foot facing forward, which is the same position as the Katakana Re.

Bogyo Gamae: Defense Stance

Bogyo Gamae means "defense posture." Here, the concern is with the position of the hands as well as the feet. The person holds the lead hand at chin level and the rear hand in front of the solar plexus. Although this is a natural stance, with the feet shoulder-width apart and the weight evenly distributed, the main aspect is a turn of the body to a 45-degree angle. The advantage of this stance is that the centerline of the body does not face the opponent.

Because most people are right-handed, the typical defense position is left foot forward, left hand at chin level, right foot at a 45-degree angle, and right hand in front of the solar plexus. But a person must be able to perform skills from the right-foot-forward stance to fight left-handed people or to defend a surprise attack from the right side.

The defense position, a staple of nearly all martial arts, is the most unobtrusive of all stances. The idea is to be ready to do anything with both hands and feet, or move into a throw or other grappling move. In Kempo, this stance offers maximum protection with minimum telegraphing, that is, alerting the attacker to one's capabilities.

Kiba Dachi: Horse Stance

The final stance assumed by the Kempoka is the horse stance. This is known as Kiba Dachi, literally the "horse-riding stance," in which the person who takes the stance looks as if he or she is riding a horse. Choki Motobu, the great Kempo master from Okinawa, always taught the use of the horse stance as the principal one for serious fighting. One usually takes the stance in a sideways fashion with the left arm and leg facing the attacker. In the horse stance the feet are twice shoulder-width apart, with the weight evenly distributed. In this position, the Kempoka can face straight forward, Mae Kiba Dachi, or at a 45-degree angle, Kakuto Kiba Dachi. Many see this as the best combat position, thus giving it the name Kakuto Kiba Dachi, or "fighting-horse stance." Finally, the practitioner can face directly sideways in a stance known as the Yoko Kiba Dachi.

From the horse stance, the person can generate great power in all strikes and kicks. When the practitioner develops proper movement in the stance, it offers a lot of stability for executing throws, joint techniques, and other grappling skills.

The horse stance is the most important stance for serious combat. The origin of this stance can be traced to the Shaolin temple, where it served as a foundation for all other techniques and was a major training posture for strengthening the legs. Kempoka of any style must have a solid horse stance and the ability to move smoothly in it, dealing with everything from hand movements to kicks.

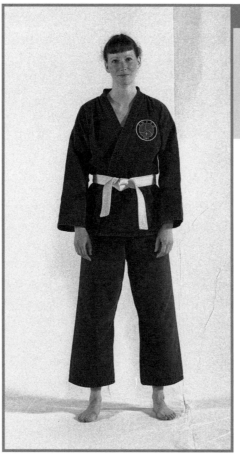

NATURAL STANCE, SHIZEN DACHI

This stance is basically the normal standing position you assume in everyday life. Your feet are shoulder-width apart, and the weight is evenly distributed between the feet. From this position, you can move in any direction in response to an attack.

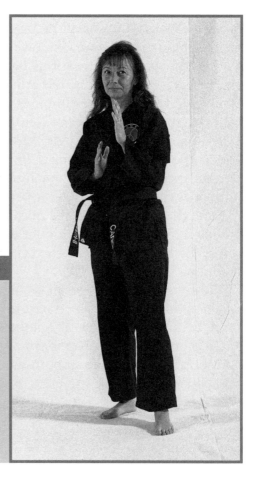

DEFENSE STANCE, BOGYO GAMAE

When you become aware of a threat, you should step back with the right foot to form a **V** shape with your feet. Your feet should still be shoulder-width apart and your weight evenly distributed, but now with your body turned 45 degrees to the right in a more protected manner. Your left hand should be in front of the chin, and your right hand should be in front of the solar plexus. This position offers maximum protection from which to begin a defensive maneuver.

HORSE STANCE, KIBA DACHI

You usually assume this stance in a sideways fashion, with the left arm and leg facing the attacker and your feet twice shoulder-width apart and parallel to one another. This position presents the least amount of target space to an assailant. Once you master this stance, you can deliver powerful strikes and kicks as well as move easily into grappling skills. Your hands may be in several postures, but the most common has the left hand high with the right arm across the solar plexus area.

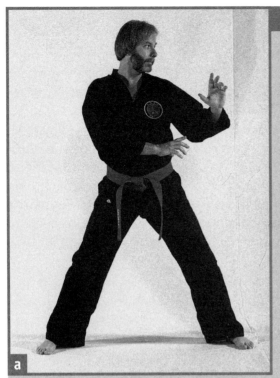

a

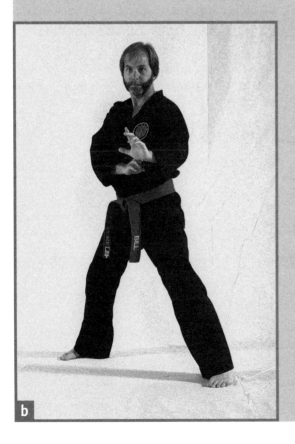

b

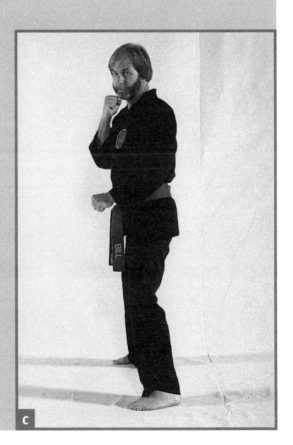

c

SECONDARY STANCES

All other stances in Kempo are transitory, positions that one moves through between the primary stances in the execution of techniques. Therefore, we can consider them secondary stances. Because the stances are transitory, the position of the hands varies according to the response necessary to an attack. The Kempoka does not always assume a particular hand position. Although students must master these stances to achieve real power and effectiveness in the execution of techniques, they must not confuse them with stances assumed in a self-defense situation. Students learn to connect them and blend them into intelligent and balanced combat footwork. Footwork, or Ashisabaki, has the feet moving from generally shoulder-width apart to about half shoulder-width apart. One must remember to move through these secondary stances, not assume them.

Leaning Back Stance

Square Back Stance

Forward Stance

Narrow Back Stance

Cat Stance

Crane Stance

Heron Stance

LEANING BACK STANCE, KEI KOKUTSU DACHI

Another special stance is effective against an attack toward the head. Lean your upper body back over the rear leg in perfect balance, using the shoulder as a blocking agent. This position allows you to kick with the lead leg or spring back with a devastating hand attack after the assault has missed.

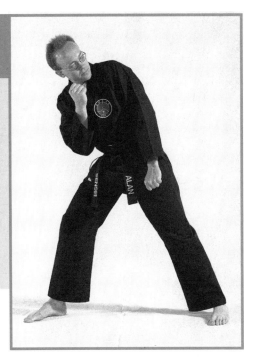

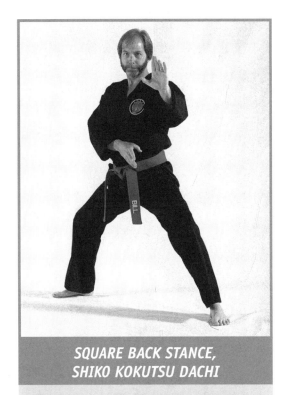

SQUARE BACK STANCE, SHIKO KOKUTSU DACHI

This stance is similar to the horse stance except that your feet are at a 90-degree angle to each other and your body is usually at a 45-degree angle to the attacker.

FORWARD STANCE, ZENKUTSU DACHI

This is the power stance of Kempo. When you want to deliver maximum power, you rotate forward from either a horse stance or a square-back stance into the forward stance. From this stance, you can strike with devastating force. It is essential that you master this stance, rotating both into it and out of it, for power and maneuverability.

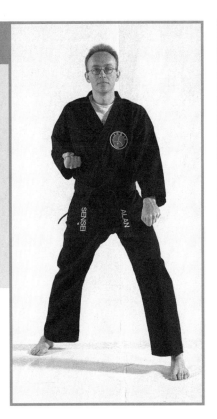

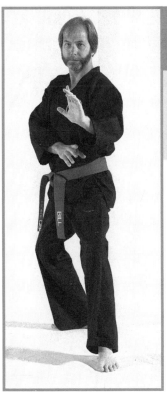

NARROW BACK STANCE, KYO KOKUTSU DACHI

You use this specialized stance for retreating, and sometimes for advancing, when in the defense position.

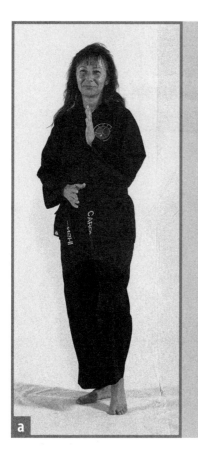

a

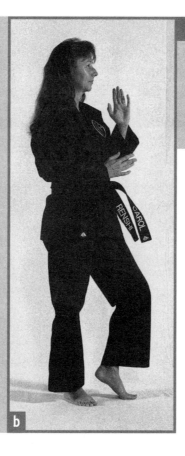

b

CAT STANCE, NEKO ASHI DACHI

In the cat-leg stance, the ball of your front foot gently touches the floor, with 90 percent of your weight on the back leg. You use this stance to prepare for kicking or, if necessary, for making a quick hop to the rear.

CRANE STANCE, TSURU ASHI DACHI

This is a one-legged stance, with the foot of the other leg resting against the side of the knee. Use this stance to prepare for kicking, usually low kicks.

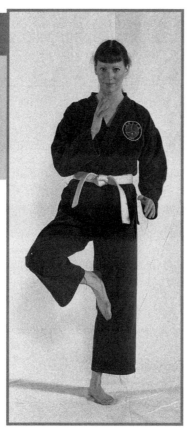

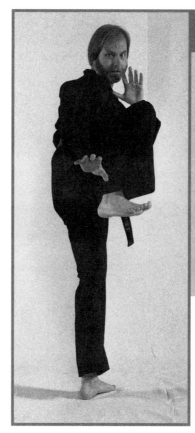

HERON STANCE, SAGI ASHI DACHI

Although some styles use only the crane stance, the heron stance is for those who have mastered Kempo kicking. For this stance, you lift your leg high with the shin perpendicular to the ground. This position provides the load for kicks waist high and above, although some stomps have devastating power from this position.

James Masayoshi Mitose (1916–1981)

Born on Hawaii, Mitose was sent to Japan at the age of five to receive a traditional education, which included the martial arts. He returned to Hawaii after studying for 15 years. When the Japanese bombed Pearl Harbor, he decided to open a school to teach Kempo to those on the Hawaiian Islands.

He retired from active teaching and moved to the continental United States in 1953. Raised a Buddhist monk, he became an ordained minister while living on the continent. In the early 1970s, he accepted a student and began to teach again.

Mitose was the first person to teach Kempo outside Japan. His style, known as Kosho Ryu, was a complete Kempo system, teaching many esoteric skills, including Karumijutsu (body-lightening art), Hayagakejutsu (fast-running art), Hichojutsu (leaping, flying, climbing art), Suieijutsu (swimming art), Koppo (bone-breaking method), and Ninjutsu (stealth art).

USING STANCES

To reach a full understanding of the use of stances, the Kempoka must comprehend the idea of movement. Kempo is nothing more than the study of motion. The Kempoka wants nothing less than to understand every possible movement of the body as well as the many different meanings of those movements.

Taisabaki: Body Movements

In the martial arts, "body movement" is pronounced Taisabaki, which refers to all possible ways that one can manipulate the body. Movements are generally broken down into two specific categories—Tesabaki and Ashisabaki.

Tesabaki: Hand Movements

Tesabaki means "hand movements" and can refer to the use of the hands and arms in the execution of blocks, strikes, punches, grabs, locks, and throws. In advanced training, Kempoka understand each movement in multiple ways so that, literally speaking, blocks are strikes, strikes are locks, and arm sweeps are throws.

Ashisabaki: Foot Movements

Ashisabaki refers to foot movements, which include not only kicks, sweeps, props, and reaps but also stances. The Okinawans in particular made a complete study of stances so that they could understand all the positions the body could find itself in while seeking stability in a fight.

The Okinawan warriors built their research on that done by Shorinji Kempo masters of China and combined it with the posture training of the Minamoto Bujutsu, martial arts from Japan. At the highest level, we hear the statement, "There are no stances in Kempo," but what that really means is that the Kempoka has trained in stances so thoroughly that he or she does them automatically, without thought, in actual combat.

In real combat, one has no time to stop and think about what the feet are supposed to do. The feet must feel what is appropriate in the environment they are in and move accordingly. This comes about only through a great deal of stance training and practice in varying environments.

Kempoka understand how important it is to practice their techniques not only in the Dojo (school) but also on the sidewalk, with shoes on, on grass, on sloping surfaces, in the house on rugs or linoleum, and in other environs where they might be attacked.

Taisabaki is thus the coordinated movement of the hands, Tesabaki, and the feet, Ashisabaki, to achieve precise motion for self-defense and survival. In self-defense, the significance of coordination is evident, but some do not recognize its value in daily survival.

We deal each day with little things that could cause injury or possibly death. We face everything from falls to low-hanging tree limbs to moving vehicles when we are pedestrians. The balance training of Taisabaki is not only about how to keep one's feet in a fight but also about how to maintain stability on a slick floor, on ice, or on a wet surface.

Although we may be called upon to block a punch in a confrontation, we cannot block a car coming at us. When a limb pushed aside by a careless person whips toward us, we will need to move as well as block.

The Kempoka have always considered Taisabaki as an aspect of dodging that is the real key to self-defense, survival, and Kempo in general. Some of the martial arts that have developed into competitive sports do not use dodging. Kempo has no specific sport form and has always emphasized dodging in combat.

Uke:
The Blocks

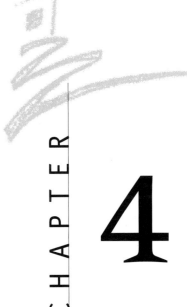

CHAPTER

4

To block actually means "to receive." Blocking has three connotations. First is the idea of the hard block, which is really a strike to the attacking limb or a blow to the assailant's body that inhibits the landing of the attack. Next is the parry, or soft block, which gently deflects the attack so that it misses. Last is the cover, in which the defender places some part of his or her limbs over the vital area that the attacker aims at. The limb rather than the vital point thus takes the hit. One should use the cover only when necessary because the blow still impacts the defender, an occurrence that is never agreeable.

Since Kempo made its way to the United States, many words have been translated in different ways. People have applied various meanings to the Japanese word Uke. Uke can be translated in all of the following ways—block, parry, catch, accept, or receive. Uke deals specifically with what to do with an opponent's attack. Kempo, originally a martial art of a religious nature, assumes that one will never attack first. This was an influence that profoundly affected the development of Karate, which has as a primary admonition, "In Karate, there is no first attack."

Therefore, in Kempo the first skill one must develop is dealing with an attacker's assault. The five translations of the term Uke give us five different methods of dealing with an attack, according to the situation. The first and most common English translation of Uke is "block."

BLOCK

Block specifically refers to stopping a blow, meeting force by force. This is the most basic method of stopping an assault. Blocking does not refer to meeting power with equal power but to going inside the point of focus, for example, blocking the forearm of a roundhouse punch.

The force of a punch is concentrated in the fist. Thus if a person is generating full power, the most dangerous point is the front of the fist, the point where all the power is generated at contact. If a Kempoka steps inside the punch, however, and blocks the forearm, he or she meets less strength so a small amount of force can stop a strong punch.

This is one of the reasons that a small person can defend himself or herself against a much larger, more powerful, attacker. The most beneficial form of blocking is to get inside the point of focus and block a weak point. If an attacker is punching, one blocks the forearm; if an attacker is kicking, one blocks the shin; if an attacker is kneeing, one blocks the thigh; and so on.

It is not always possible to get inside a blow, so the Kempoka might need to cover the vital point being targeted and accept the strike on a strong part of the body. For example, if someone is trying to hit you in the ribs, you might pull the upper arm into position to cover them, taking the hit on the arm rather than on the vulnerable ribs. This is the least favorable strategy of blocking but one that all Kempoka must be able to use when no other option is workable.

PARRY

The second aspect of Uke is to parry. A parry is the deflection of an attack to a different axis, which causes it to miss its intended target. A second benefit of using a parry is that because the attack misses its target, the assailant generally ends up in an unbalanced position. This circumstance offers the defender a better opportunity to control or defeat the attacker.

Parries are most efficient against linear attacks, although a skillful Kempoka can apply them against certain circular techniques. Parries are more advanced skills than blocks and indicate a much higher level of ability.

CATCH

The next aspect of Uke is to catch. This progressive skill develops from the parry. The catch deals with how to grab an attacker's limb or body in a defensive manner, allowing the defender to control or throw the attacker. Superior skill is required to catch an assailant in the midst of an attack and then pin or throw the person with the force the attacker has generated.

ACCEPT

The next phase of Uke is to accept, the idea of blending with the energy of the attacker. This is where the concept of Aiki derives from its Kempo roots. When an attacker moves to strike or grapple an advanced Kempoka, the martial artist blends with the movement, captures the energy, and uses it to spiral the opponent away or into submission.

These four aspects of Uke are generally taught with the specific movements of the outer circular block and the inner circular block, which one can apply in all four manners. These are the most important blocks of Kempo and form the foundation of nearly all other blocks and parries. It is essential that the student master these two blocks at the outset of Kempo training, for this will make learning the advanced skills much easier.

RECEIVE

The last aspect of this important Kempo principle is to receive. We can use the term generically to encompass any method of "receiving" an attack, but in the advanced levels, receiving refers to moving in such a way that the assault cannot disturb the Kempoka's center. In many situations, the practitioner simply uses a dodge so that a strike or grab misses. Under other circumstances, he or she uses a body shift that takes the body out of alignment with the attacker so that the person cannot make contact with the defender.

Receiving has always been considered the highest level of skill. This ability to outmaneuver an opponent through superior body movement is often referred to as Taisabaki. This facet of Kempo affects the application of all

William Chow (1914–1987)

Chow studied many forms of martial arts, the most prominent being Kosho Ryu Kempo under James Mitose. He blended Kosho Ryu Kempo with Shaolinssu Chuanfa (Shorinji Kempo) to form his own style, now known as Kara Ho Kempo Karate.

Chow was known as an excellent and powerful martial artist. He opened his first school in 1944, emphasizing the Karate aspect of Kempo in his teachings. Chow taught many excellent martial artists in his time, the most famous of whom was Ed Parker.

other skills because the movement that evades an attack allows the practitioner to be in position to apply a counter, either a strike or a throw.

Generally, to make a defense safer, one combines two or more of these moves. For example, a Kempoka may evade and parry, or block and catch. In the execution of certain connected techniques, one might even combine a dodge, a block, and a catch.

An important term concerning blocking is Kaihi, which can be translated simply as "dodge" but carries with it the idea of combination. Kai can mean "go around," and Hi means "ward off." Both concepts should be a normal part of blocking. Even a highly skilled person might miss a block, but if he or she has dodged as well, the hit will not connect.

Also, it may be impossible to block at times, such as when the hands are full, but those accustomed to dodging and blocking will still have a defense. In other circumstances, a person may be unable to dodge, such as when an assailant attacks in a hallway. A Kempoka must then have excellent blocking skills. Thus as one learns how to block, he or she should also learn how to dodge in coordination with the blocking movements.

English-speaking Kempoka will simply use the word blocks for the techniques of defense. But there is much more to the blocking techniques of Kempo than we generally attribute to the word block. Regardless of terminology, someone wishing to reach the highest levels of Kempo must master all five aspects of Uke.

Outer Circular Block

Inner Circular Block

Cross Block

X Block

Rising Block

Inside Forearm Block

Outside Forearm Block

Downward Block

Tiger Claw Catch

Wing Block

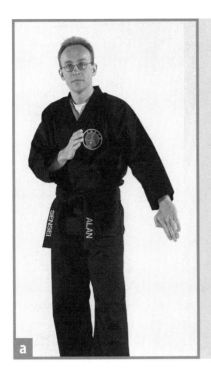

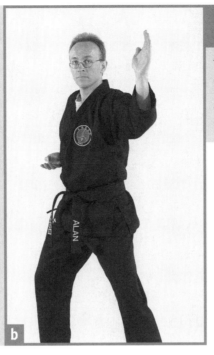

OUTER CIRCULAR BLOCK, SOTO MAWASHI UKE

This block can trace a complete 360-degree circle, but you usually use it to block a punch or strike directed at your head, which means that the first quarter of movement stops the incoming blow.

INNER CIRCULAR BLOCK, UCHI MAWASHI UKE

This block also describes a 360-degree circle. You most commonly use it to block low blows and kicks.

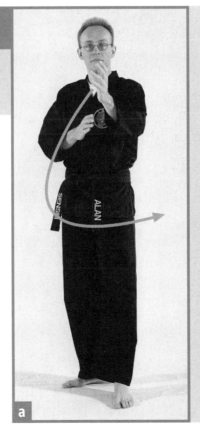

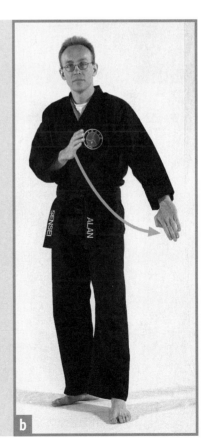

CROSS BLOCK, YOKOGIRU UKE

Move the hand that starts at the shoulder and travels across the body to parry, or hard-block, a blow coming at the chest or face.

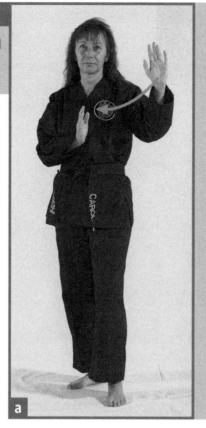

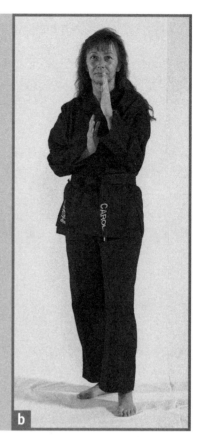

X BLOCK, JUJI UKE

Cross the forearms to form a wedge in which to catch an attacker's limb. Although you usually use the **X** block in an upper position to catch downward blows, you can orient it downward to catch frontal kicks.

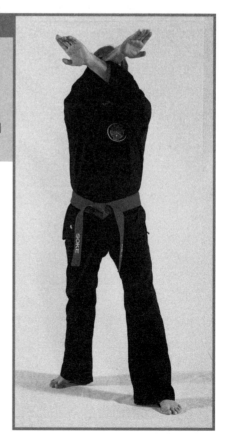

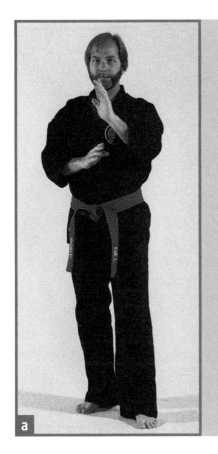

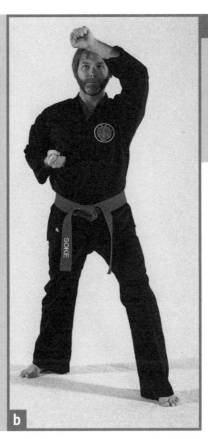

RISING BLOCK, AGE UKE

Bring the forearm upward in a direct manner to hard-block and parry a linear attack from underneath, or to hard-block and parry a descending blow by using a diagonal angle. The rising block must be 45 degrees in relation to the face to deflect a downward blow.

a

b

INSIDE FOREARM BLOCK, UCHI UDE UKE

Use the thumb side of the forearm to deflect to the outside of the body a punch directed at the chest. Perform this with a forearm twist to add power and deflection to the block.

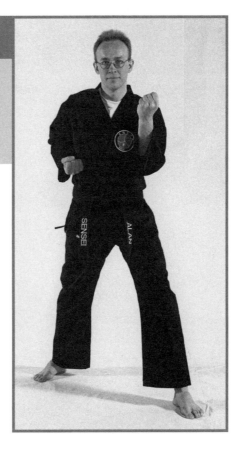

OUTSIDE FOREARM BLOCK, SOTO UDE UKE

Use the little-finger side of the forearm to deflect a punch directed at the chest, across the body and away.

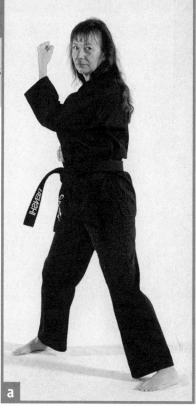

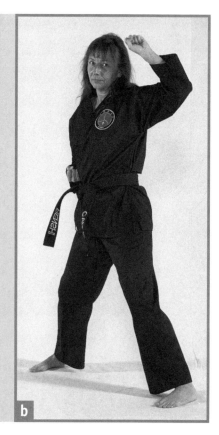

DOWNWARD BLOCK, GEDAN UKE

The downward block is a powerful and damaging block for any technique directed at the stomach. Your arm starts at the shoulder of the opposite arm and traces a circle down across the stomach.

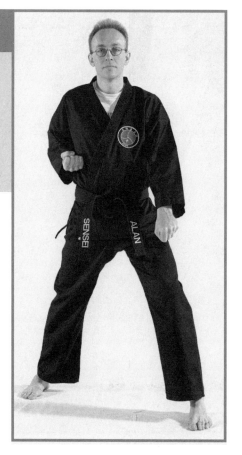

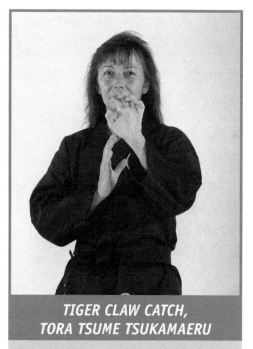

TIGER CLAW CATCH, TORA TSUME TSUKAMAERU

In practice, the tiger claw catch strengthens your forearm because of dynamic tension, but in application, the claw conforms to the fist of the attacker. It is essential to catch the attacker's punch early in its execution before it develops maximum force. Your arm must extend more than 90 degrees.

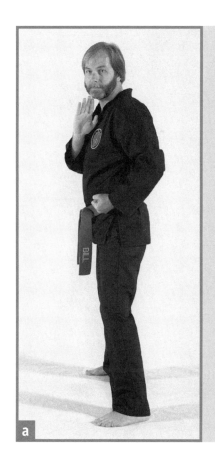
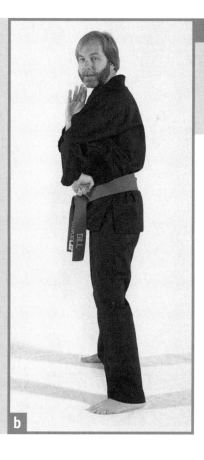

WING BLOCK, HANE UKE

This relaxed, parrying form of block deflects anything directed to the ribs with an outward swing of the arm. Done properly, this block protects from the waist all the way up to the shoulder.

Blocking is such an essential part of self-defense that it does not seem necessary to defend the concept. But people have begun to think of blocking as unnecessary, unusable, and impractical since the martial arts have come to the West and developed into rough-and-tumble forms of combat. This false idea has developed from the introduction of Western boxing techniques into full- and light-contact forms of fighting in which fighters attack hesitantly and with snappy blows that are too quick to catch or block. But most people who advocate abandoning blocking as a fighting skill are unaware that people do not box in real-life fights.

Tsuki:
The Thrusts

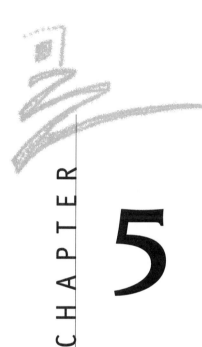

CHAPTER

5

Thrusts, known as Tsuki, can be performed in many ways. When done with the fist, the techniques are driven straight forward, generally smashing into the target with the forefist, the first two knuckles.

Tsuki is another Japanese word that can have various meanings. It also has two distinct meanings in English according to which style of Kempo you choose.

In the least correct usage of the term, Tsuki has been translated as "punch." Any technique using the fist is thus called a Tsuki, regardless of whether the fist takes a straight or circular path.

In several Karate styles, Tsuki is translated mainly as "thrust," meaning that only those techniques that travel a straight line are Tsuki. In this context, punches, fingertip strikes, heel-palm blows, or any other hand technique that follows a straight line are Tsuki.

Tsuki actually translates to "thrust, spear, stab, poke, and strike." With such a range of meaning, any of the interpretations discussed earlier is correct. In the typical Japanese sense, however, the meaning "movement in a straight line" is most correct.

In Kempo systems that do not use the Japanese language, the techniques are referred to simply as punches or strikes. Punches are the techniques of the fist, whereas strikes are performed with the open hand or other parts of the body, such as elbows, shoulders, hips, and others, excluding the legs.

TYPES OF THRUSTS

This manual will include the various thrusts as interpreted in the Japanese manner. The hand or fist can be loaded in many different ways, allowing movement in a relatively straight line to its intended target. I use the word relatively because any human movement tends to trace a slight arc.

Tsuki: Thrust

The main punch in many styles of Kempo is often called simply Tsuki, or thrust. The Kempoka generally practices it with the fist starting at the side of the body, with the palm up. The person then punches the fist forward, turning to the palm-down position after the elbow has passed the side of the body. This punch is also the primary punch of most Karate styles.

Tate Tsuki: Vertical Fist

Some Kempo systems have as their primary punch a vertical fist technique that does not twist or rotate. The twisting punch reflects an Okinawan influence, whereas the punch without a twist has a Japanese influence. Note that regardless of whether the punch twists or not, punching in Kempo is extremely powerful because it comes from the mind.

I Ken: The Mind

One of the Chinese influences on Okinawan martial arts is a style named I Chuan, or in Japanese, I Ken. This translates as "will fist," referring to the fact that the mind directs the power of the punch. One punches not only with the power of the body but also with the power of the mind. When one understands that intent directs Ki, the spiritual, internal strength inherent in the human being (a primary principle of Tai Chi Chuan, another Chinese art influential on Okinawan styles of Kempo), then one recognizes that the power of the Kempo punch is phenomenal.

Nukite: Spear Hands

Other thrusts of Kempo are those performed with Nukite, the "spear hands," which include the one-finger spear, two-finger spear, four-finger spear, and the spear hand. The heel palm is also a thrusting technique as are the inverted punch, jab, leopard fist, leopard paw, twin dragon, and others. The Kempoka must realize that the thrusts should hit a target with a 90-degree intersection to exert maximum power into the vital point. Again, note that Kempoka never hit in a general manner but always seek to strike vulnerable areas or pressure points on an opponent's body for maximum effect.

The shortest distance between two points is a straight line. Thus whenever an opportunity to travel a straight line to a target is available, the practitioner takes it. In general, thrusts are directed to three levels, designated high, middle, and low. In combat, high usually refers to thrusts directed at the head, middle to torso thrusts, and low to thrusts directed below the waist.

In many ways, the linear technique is the easiest to defend against, so Kempo is rich in circular techniques, the topic of the next chapter.

Twisting Punch

Vertical Punch

Inverted Punch

Jab

Leopard Fist Punch

Spear Hand

Four-Finger Spear

Two-Finger Spear

One-Finger Spear

Twin Dragon

Heel Palm

Leopard Paw

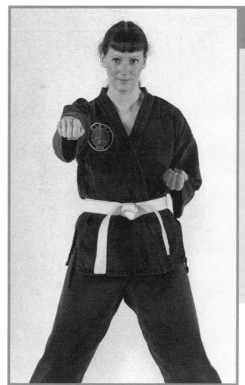

TWISTING PUNCH, TSUKI

Commonly called simply the thrust, this is the typical punch of Kempo and Karate. The technique starts with the punch held palm up at the side. You execute it by bringing the punch from the side to the front. Proper Kempo form requires you to launch the punch straight off the shoulder, focusing on hitting with just the first two knuckles of the fist.

VERTICAL PUNCH, TATE TSUKI

This thrust is similar to the twisting punch, but the fist does not travel as far forward and it stops in the vertical position. You therefore use the vertical punch for shorter range fighting, but it is still a two-knuckle fist strike.

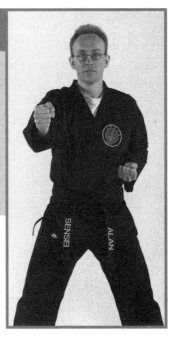

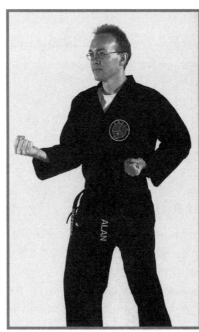

INVERTED PUNCH, SAKASA TSUKI

You use this punch when very close to an opponent. It is a two-knuckle punch directed to the ribs or other Kyusho on the torso. The punch stays palm up during the entire technique.

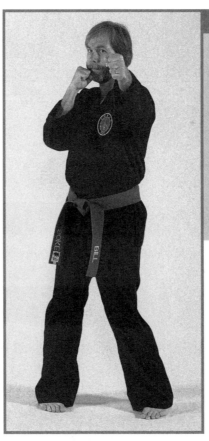

JAB, SOKU TSUKI

The Kempo jab is different from a boxer's jab, which actually has more in common with the twisting punch. You perform the Kempo jab in a Sanchin stance using body rotation to throw your whole body behind the punch. Snap the jab out and back quickly, using a vertical fist.

LEOPARD FIST PUNCH, HYOKEN TSUKI

The leopard fist differs from the standard fist in its formation. The thumb, instead of being cocked across the fingers, is locked on top of the fingers. In the thrust, you use the two knuckles of the forefist for striking in all the ways mentioned earlier. As we will see, however, this is but one of the weapons of the Hyoken.

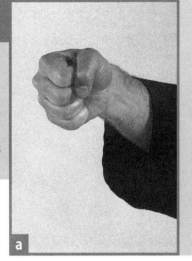

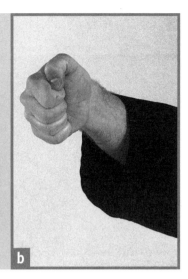

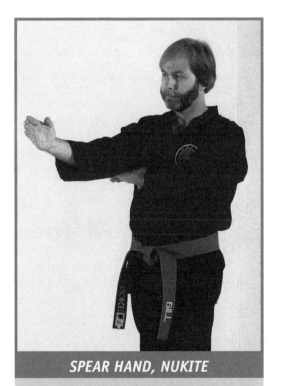

SPEAR HAND, NUKITE

By cocking the thumb, the hand becomes as strong as it can be. Over the years, through dynamic tension, it will become incredibly strong. You perform the spear hand with the fingertips held together and aimed only at soft vital points.

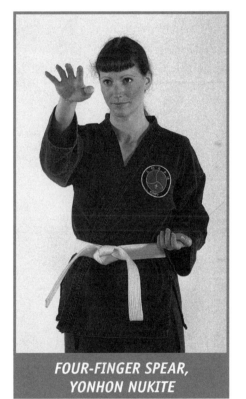

FOUR-FINGER SPEAR, YONHON NUKITE

In this technique, the fingers are separated and normally aimed at the eyes so that at least one or two fingers will strike the target.

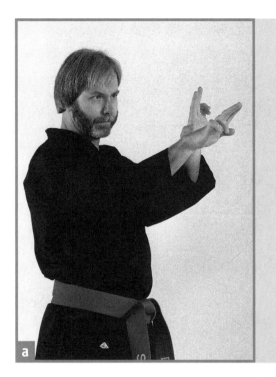

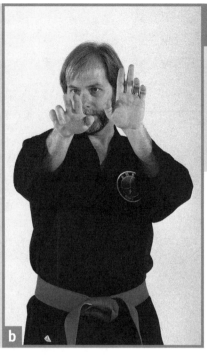

TWO-FINGER SPEAR, NIHON NUKITE

A person who has great speed and accuracy can use the two-finger spear. Again, the eyes are the normal target, although one who has spent years in training will be able to strike other vital points effectively.

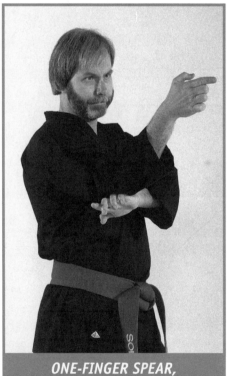

ONE-FINGER SPEAR, IPPON NUKITE

A person who has developed great strength in the hands can use one finger to strike a number of vital points effectively and accurately.

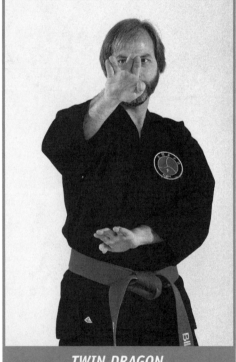

TWIN DRAGON, SO RYU

This technique is stronger than the one-finger spear, so it is suitable for the beginner to use when striking the eyes. The advanced practitioner can use it to damage other vital points, especially those in the throat.

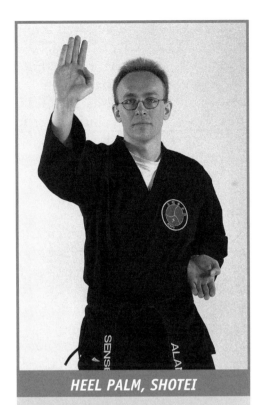

HEEL PALM, SHOTEI

This technique uses the bottom of the hand near the wrist, with the hand flexed back, to strike with a linear thrust.

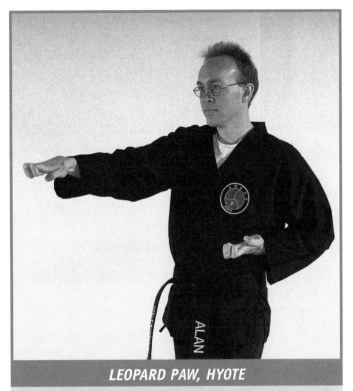

LEOPARD PAW, HYOTE

This technique is sometimes referred to as Hiraken, the flat fist. With it, you strike with the extended knuckles. You should use the leopard paw only to strike soft vital points because this area of the hand is not as strong as the forefist area. This technique causes maximum damage, however, when used on an appropriate Kyusho.

TEKKEN: IRON FIST

A great legend to come out of China tells of Chugoku Kempo masters who possessed an iron fist that could strike an opponent with the force of a mace. Those stories traveled with the martial arts to Japan and Okinawa. Many tried to figure out how the Chinese masters could generate such a weapon, and they sought to develop their own ways of creating the iron fist.

One method that the Kempo masters of China, Japan, and Okinawa used was to strike their fists and hands against progressively harder substances. They started with buckets of sand, progressed to small rocks, and then advanced to slightly larger rocks. By striking against these rocks, the hands became hard and strong.

Other Kempoka punched bundles of straw, then bundles of sticks, and finally wooden slabs. A few masters tried punching boulders, cliff walls, and even metal anvils or slabs of metal. Those who adhere to this type of training claim the fist will become as hard as the substances it strikes against. It is true that hard calluses will form on the fist and that the layers of the skin will thicken wherever struck against hard surfaces.

The main problem with this type of training is that although one may develop a truly devastating punch, the hands suffer damage and may lose some sensitivity and dexterity. The hands become less capable of movement at advanced stages and can develop serious problems like arthritis.

The second way that the iron fist was purportedly developed was more esoteric. Ki has always been considered the most important principle in the training of the martial arts, figuring in many uses and applications. In regard to Tekken, the "iron fist," it was thought that a person could focus Ki into the hand in such a way that without much conditioning it would become like an object of iron.

In the 1970s, a movie released in the United States called *The Five Fingers of Death* dealt with the legend of the iron fist. The movie portrayed the might of the iron fist by having the hands of the martial artist glow when he invoked its power. What was funny was that people took seriously the image of the gleaming iron fist. I remember talking to a person training in a martial-arts form who said that the movie revealed secrets of the martial arts that were never intended for the public. It was laughable.

Although Ki does in fact empower martial-arts techniques, never has a master started glowing in public. This kind of fantasy must be kept in check if the martial arts are to progress.

A secret of Tekken has indeed existed, passed from master to master and kept from less dedicated students or potentially violent ones. In that way, students who might abuse the power of the martial arts would waste their time in the fantasy pursuit of glowing, or would damage themselves smashing their bodies against various hard surfaces.

I will now reveal, for the first time in print, the real secret of the Tekken. The secret of the iron fist is to direct your blows always to the weakest part of an opponent's anatomy so that your fist is like iron compared with what it hits. As So Doshin, the founder of Nippon Shorinji Kempo, put it, the human body was made strong enough to defend itself; one simply must learn how to use it correctly.

Tekken is to take the fist, hand, or any bodily weapon and apply it against the Kyusho, the vital points. Thus the real secret of Tekken, the iron fist of legend, is to strike effectively at the most fragile part of the opponent's body.

KYUSHO

Kyusho are the points that strikes and grappling techniques can damage. Kyusho comprises three major divisions.

The primary vital points are the eyes, throat, and groin. In gravely threatening situations, these are the main targets, but one should attack these points only if there is no recourse. When a person's life is on the line, however, he or she should target those points with vigor.

The secondary vital points are other areas where a strike or grappling technique can cause injury. These include the solar plexus, mastoid process, and the like, as well as the major joints of the body and the weak areas of the skeletal structure.

Finally, the third set of vital points are those connected to acupuncture, or Shinjutsu, and acupressure, or Shiatsu. The proper use of these vital points is extremely difficult to master. Advanced Kempoka and other advanced martial artists should study them academically. All should remember, however, that the primary and secondary points are the indispensable elements to everyday self-defense.

Figures 5.1 and 5.2 show the main vital points from the first two categories. Every Kempoka should be able to target them at will in actual movement, practicing especially in Kihon Kumite, Renzoku Ken, and Embu.

Primary Targets

The art of Kempo has always been the art of the underdog, a way for a person weaker than an opponent or outnumbered by a gang to equalize the odds. One cannot accomplish this without having something significant to balance the scales. This is where the study of Kyusho comes into play.

It is not enough to know how to hit and kick well. One must be sure to execute effective strikes. This begins by knowing where to hit an assailant to maximize the effect of the hit. A hit or kick to some targets will devastate an opponent. A strike to other targets will stun or incapacitate, without causing injury or death.

In dangerous confrontations, the three primary targets are the eyes, throat, and groin. If one strikes any of these three areas correctly, the blow will disable the attacker.

Eyes

The eyes can be struck in three different manners. Light taps will cause watering, blurred vision, and disorientation. Hard pressure can severely injure the eyeball or cause it to rupture, which can lead to permanent blindness or limited vision. Finally, the eye can be raked, which can cause serious eye problems by scratching, tearing, or scarring the cornea or iris.

Throat

An attack on the throat can collapse the trachea or crush the larynx. If the trachea is collapsed by a blow, a healthy throat will spring back, with the effect being disorientation, pain, and gagging. If, however, the throat is unhealthy because of heavy smoking and drinking, it can be fragile. When it collapses, it cracks on the inside, causing bleeding into the lungs. Swelling may also occur, which can close off the windpipe.

A crushed larynx usually does not cause life-threatening effects, but the larynx itself will be irreparable. The person may lose the ability to speak or may speak only with a heavily, often negatively, modified voice.

Groin

The groin has always been regarded as the ultimate target on males, but one should not overvalue the effect of a strike there. Many men can take strong hits to that area and keep fighting. Some psychotics enjoy the pain of a strike there, becoming more aroused toward rape or brutalizing women.

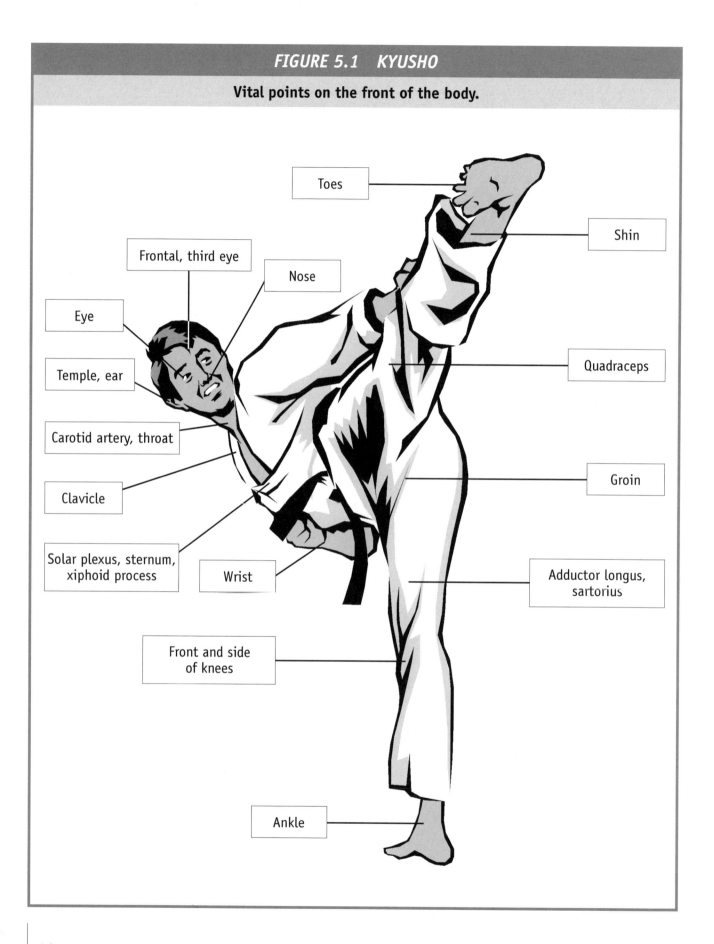

FIGURE 5.1   KYUSHO

Vital points on the front of the body.

Toes

Shin

Frontal, third eye

Nose

Eye

Quadraceps

Temple, ear

Carotid artery, throat

Groin

Clavicle

Solar plexus, sternum, xiphoid process

Wrist

Adductor longus, sartorius

Front and side of knees

Ankle

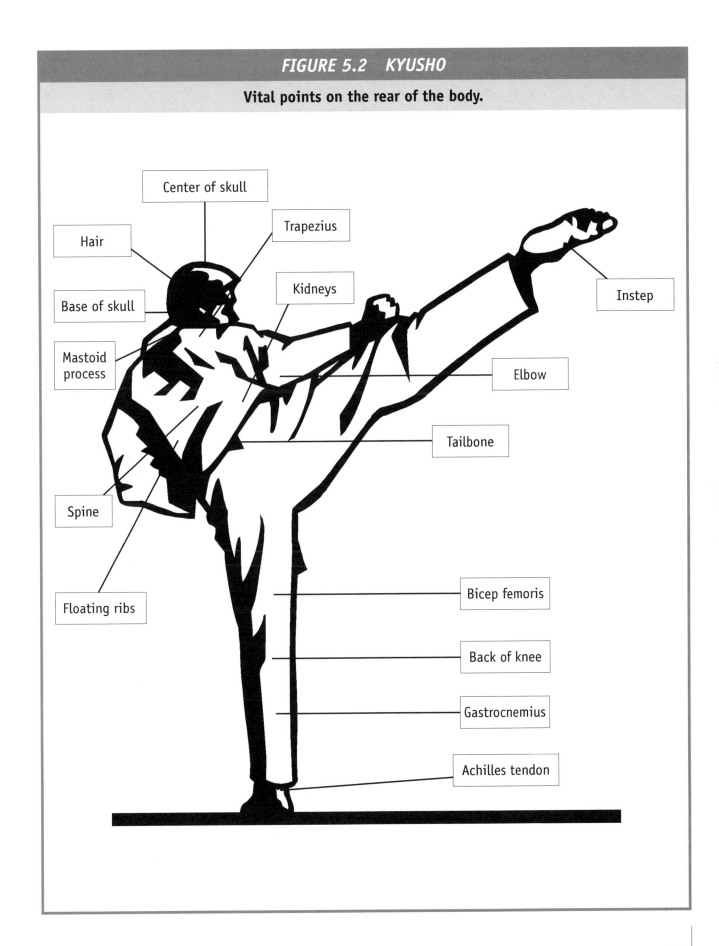

FIGURE 5.2   KYUSHO

Vital points on the rear of the body.

Center of skull

Trapezius

Hair

Kidneys

Base of skull

Instep

Mastoid process

Elbow

Tailbone

Spine

Bicep femoris

Floating ribs

Back of knee

Gastrocnemius

Achilles tendon

When one targets the groin, it should be with the idea of hitting a testicle with force sufficient to cause severe compression, which can possibly knock a person out. The idea is to get the gonad in a location where it is compressed between the weapon one is using and the pelvic bone.

Another good strategy when attacking the groin is to grab, squeeze, and twist with as much force as one can muster. This method has been known to make a rapist helpless when the victim had the tenacity to grab and hang on for as long as it took to take the attacker down. Men have passed out from this type of defense.

Finally, in menacing situations, the goal of a strike to the groin is to cause a testicle to rupture. When this happens, a determined fighter can go on fighting for a time, but eventually the pain will become too intense. The internal bleeding caused by the rupture will end the fight.

It is obvious that one should strike these target areas only in life-threatening situations when the failure to inflict serious injury or otherwise disable the attacker will lead to one's own serious injury or death, or the injury or death of an innocent.

The problem with targeting the three vital points is that everyone knows what they are and will protect them. A good fighter with a lot of experience in the street will protect those areas as effectively as an experienced martial artist will. The person training for self-defense must therefore know the larger list of secondary targets.

Secondary Targets

Blows to secondary targets can cause extreme pain and serious injury. The student should review each of these points under a qualified instructor and learn where they are located, how to hit them, and what effect a strike will cause. The Kempoka should memorize these points for serious use in self-defense:

1. Center or top of head	11. Knees
2. Ears	12. Shin
3. Mastoid process	13. Instep
4. Nose	14. Toes
5. Chin	15. Base of skull
6. Collarbone	16. Top of spine
7. Lower third of sternum	17. Anywhere along the spine
8. Solar plexus	18. Kidneys
9. Floating ribs	19. Tailbone
10. Bladder	20. Elbows

When targeting the knees and elbows, one should understand that the joints must be straight for the blow to achieve the desired effect. Bent knees and elbows are very strong and make excellent weapons, but when these joints are straight, only a little pressure can dislocate them. Serious injury to

Ed Parker (1931–1990)

Parker studied Kempo under William Chow on Hawaii. Parker moved to the continent to attend Brigham Young University in 1951. After graduating, Parker moved to Pasadena, California, where he opened a Kempo Karate school.

Parker is celebrated as the instructor to movie stars, among them Elvis Presley, Robert Wagner, McDonald Carey, Robert Culp, Darrin McGavin, George Hamilton, Warren Beatty, Robert Conrad, Fabian, Dick Martin, Elke Summers, Joey Bishop, Nick Adams, and Audie Murphy. Parker appeared in several movies and television shows, gave hundreds of demonstrations, and wrote many books.

ligaments, tendons, and muscles usually results from a blow to a straight joint. A joint that has sustained damage will generally never be quite the same, usually suffering some loss in mobility and agility.

Tertiary Targets

We must address two final groups of vital points: (a) the muscle insertions and Tsubo, hollow points of the body, and (b) the Shiatsu, finger pressure points, which are the Shinjutsu, acupuncture points.

Tsubo: Hollow Places

The Tsubo refer to places on the body that open into hollow areas of the body. Punches that land in such places, those not covered by bone or thick layers of muscles, will more easily cause internal damage. Study of an anatomy chart will reveal these points to a person interested enough to seek them out. Muscle insertions, which one can also locate on an anatomy chart, are the areas where muscles connect to bone. These points are susceptible to injury, especially when they receive a strike or when a limb twists beyond the range of its natural movement.

Shiatsu: Pressure Points

Some people study acupressure or acupuncture charts with the hope of discovering secret places that one might hit to render a person unconscious or to kill with a touch. As mentioned earlier, the concept of the delayed death touch is more fantasy than reality. Study of these charts, however, can identify points that one can strike with notable effect. Note that many of these points correspond to the vital points mentioned earlier or are located along the routes of major blood vessels and follow the path of the nerves.

As one Okinawan master put it, nerves are found everywhere on the human body. Hit one sufficiently and you will cause some pain or damage. Overload the nervous system with enough pain and you will cause unconsciousness.

Uchi: The Strikes

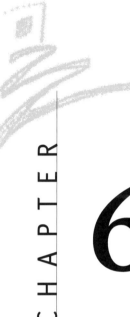

Uchi, or strikes, are techniques that travel in a circular path. Some strikes make use of stealth concepts, reaching into a vital point before an assailant knows it has been targeted. The most important aspect of fist strikes is that they hit hard with a great deal of centrifugal force. One point to keep in mind is that the circular motion is easier to see, hence easier to intercept, than the straight thrusts. With training, however, a good Kempoka can use circular techniques at the right moment to overcome this deficiency.

Uchi is commonly translated as "strike," although, like most Japanese terms, it has a more varied meaning. Literally, Uchi can mean "strike, hit, beat, slap, and punch." Given this range of meaning, some have used the term to stand for any type of blow, including straight-line punching. Specifically, however, we apply Uchi to any technique that traces a circular movement in the air.

Others have used strike to mean any blow performed with the open hand or other body part except the fists or feet. Again looking at the Japanese for an understanding of the terminology, we see that the most proper use is for circular hitting, whether with a fist or an open-hand technique.

Strikes, as circular techniques, come in a variety of styles. The Shaolin influence contributes the five animal skills—the leopard, crane, tiger, snake, and dragon—as well as other types of circular techniques. From this source also come the grappling skills of Kempo, which range from throws to joint locks and even chokes.

Circular skills are so varied that they can be strikes one minute and grappling moves the next. Depending on which historical concept one accepts, grappling skills are derived from either the dragon techniques of Shorinji Kempo or the crane techniques of southern Hakutsuru Kempo, the white-crane fist law.

Probably both Chinese Kempo styles, as well as the Torite of Japan and other grappling Bujutsu of the Samurai, influenced Okinawan development. Most, if not all, of the grappling skills of Kempo are based on the use of circular motion to break balance, disrupt physical alignment, and entrap by wrapping, all of which lead to superior throwing and grappling skills.

CIRCULAR TECHNIQUES

As strikes, the circular movements are among the most effective and diverse skills of Kempo. The hands can be open, claws, fists, or other more specialized formations. Like thrusts, which one can perform at three levels, strikes can be performed in several ways. Here we have eight angles through which each of the various strikes can travel. The practitioner can also blend several angles into one smooth movement to create comprehensive combinations so fluid and inexorable that a less experienced opponent will find them nearly impossible to counter.

By combining linear techniques with circular ones, the practitioner can attain phenomenal potential for overwhelming an attacker. When one practices Kempo as it was originally created, with no set patterns but instead with a comprehensive understanding of the principles that permit a spontaneous blending of movement to meet any situation, then the number of Kempo techniques becomes infinite.

Many martial arts teach the centerline theory of combat, emphasizing attacks on the centerline because it is the most vulnerable area of the body. Yet when we study the Kyusho of the human body, we realize that no matter how someone aligns with an opponent, someplace is vulnerable to a strike.

The circular techniques can go around, over, and under many defenses, and the linear skills can drive straight to any vital point that an assailant exposes by reacting to the strikes. The circular techniques create much of the advanced strategy of Kempo. Styles that limit themselves to an emphasis on linear movements miss the greatest range of Kempo skills.

The leading striking techniques of Kempo are the back fists and knife-hand techniques, commonly called chops. The Kempoka can apply many other strikes with various hand formations, as well as the grappling skills previously mentioned.

Some people have misunderstood Mitose's teachings on Kempo, believing that he did not include circular techniques in his art. But people outside his system who were not allowed to view his teaching made these observations. Actually, Mitose taught a full range of circular skills based on his Jujutsu experience.

The most amazing aspect of Kempo striking is its versatility, which will be demonstrated in the chapter on Renzoku Ken.

Fist Strikes	**Open-Hand Strikes**
Back Fist	*Knife Hand*
Hammer Fist	*Reverse Knife Hand*
Thumb Knuckle Strike	*Slap*
Flare Punch	*Tiger Claw*
Hook Punch	*Back Hand*
	Crane's Beak
	Bent Wrist

Fist Strikes

Some circular strikes are executed using a fist. Such strikes can be devastating, and the practitioner can use them effectively on most parts of the body.

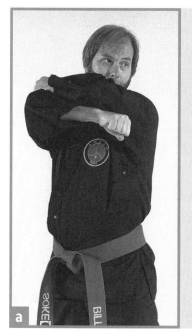
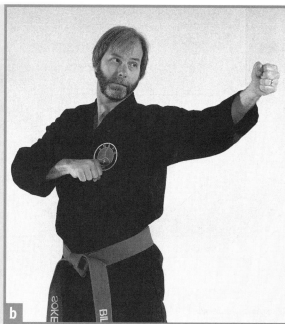

BACK FIST, URAKEN

Some feel that the back fist is the signature technique of Kempo. It is quick, powerful, and deceptive, which means that it can get in and hit vital points with the back of the forefist knuckles before an opponent can see it coming.

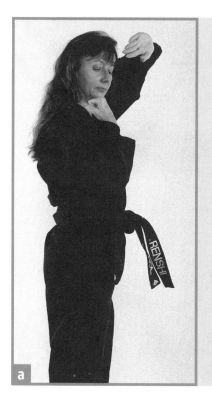
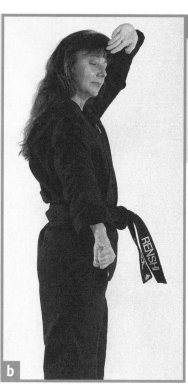

HAMMER FIST, KENTSUI

With this technique, you hit with the bottom of the fist, swinging it like a hammer. You can use the hammer fist from any angle. Hence, it can be deceiving and extremely powerful. The photograph portrays the low hammer fist aimed at the groin and offers an example of the deceptiveness of Kempo striking.

THUMB KNUCKLE STRIKE, OYAYUBI UCHI

The thumb knuckle is a part of the Hyoken, leopard fist, and uses the joint of the thumb to hit, or press, into nerve centers. You bring it into play in a circular manner, from any angle.

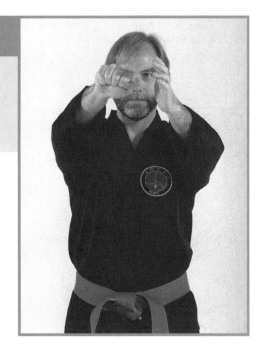

FLARE PUNCH, FURI KEN UCHI

This special, deceptive punch uses a swing of the elbow to circle the back knuckles of the fist into vital points, especially those on the head and neck.

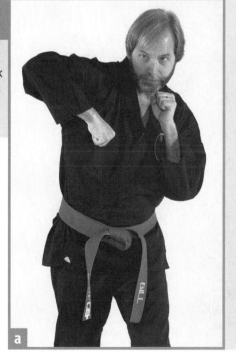

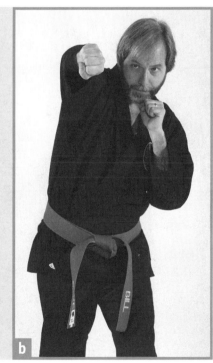

HOOK PUNCH, KAGI KEN UCHI

The Kempo hook punch is similar to a boxing hook except that it emphasizes use of the pectoral muscles to increase the power of the punch. Thus a good hook ends up bent 90 degrees at the elbow and shoulder, making it an extremely powerful technique at close range.

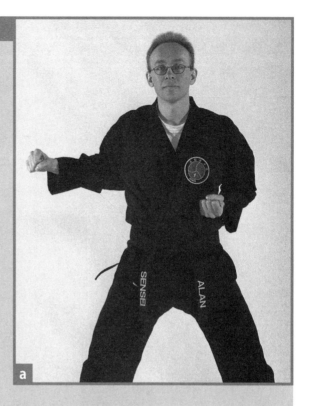

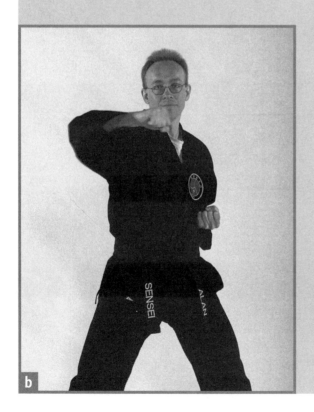

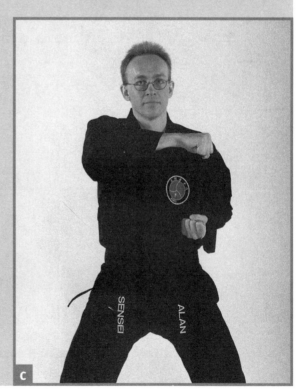

Open-Hand Strikes

Kempo is most famous for the many strikes that its practitioners can perform with the open hand, many of which are related to the various animals derived from the Shaolin temple. These specialized strikes hit deep into vital points, damaging nerves and internal organs as well as blood vessels. The circular movements are the pinnacle of Chinese Kempo styles and greatly influenced the Kempo of Okinawa and, through there, the Kempo of Japan.

KNIFE HAND, SHUTO

The knife hand, also a crane technique, uses the edge of the hand circularly from the outside to the inside. You generally aim it at the neck to compress nerves and blood vessels.

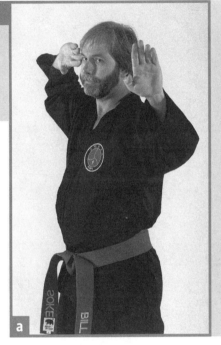
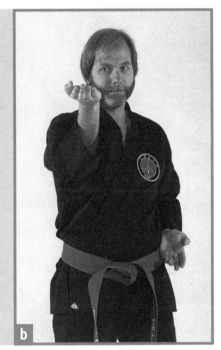

REVERSE KNIFE HAND, GYAKU SHUTO

This technique, one of the crane techniques, is an inside-to-outside movement. To perform it, you hit with the edge of the hand above the wrist and below the little finger.

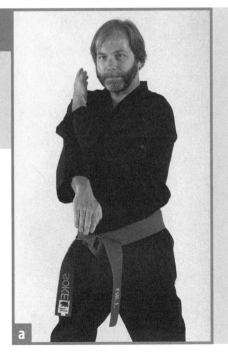
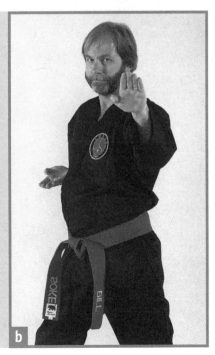

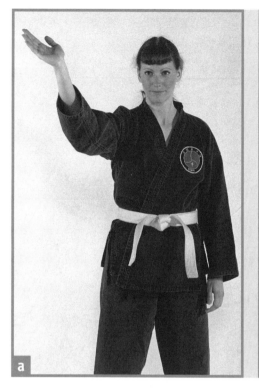 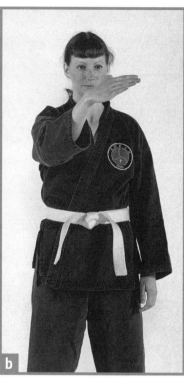

a

b

SLAP, HIRATE UCHI

Although most people think they know how to slap, this technique is not the standard sting-the-face hit. To generate power, perform the slap with focus on the lower area of the hand and the rotation of your body.

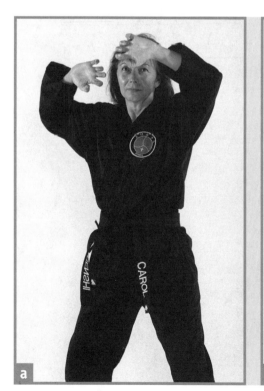 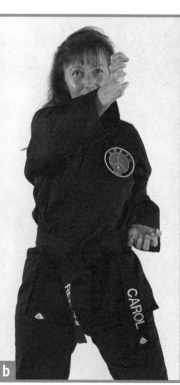

a

b

TIGER CLAW, TORA TSUME

This technique is also known as Koken, the "tiger fist." You hit with the heel of the hand and then, when appropriate, rip and tear with your fingers, which you have curled into the claw position. The raking of the tiger claw can mark an assailant for police recognition or open the forehead so that blood gets into the eyes.

BACK HAND, HAISHU

You can use the back of your hand to deliver a powerful, nonlethal strike that can knock an assailant off the feet or set the assailant up for a throw of some sort.

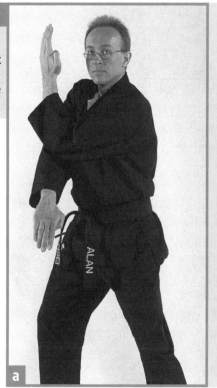

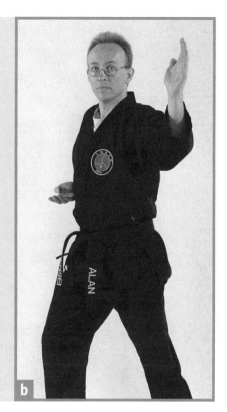

CRANE'S BEAK, TSURU KUCHIBASHI

This technique uses the joined fingers, which can also be called Kakushi, still meaning crane's beak. You can use this technique to strike vital points with devastating effect.

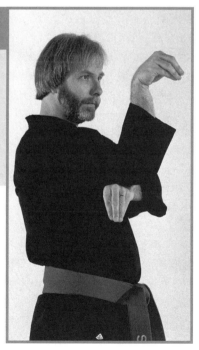

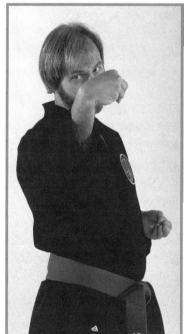

BENT WRIST, KAKUTO

The bent wrist, considered a part of the crane techniques, is useful for close-in, surprise strikes. You bend the wrist forward and use it to strike soft areas of the body, with surprising impact.

UCHITE: HITTING

In the study of the Okinawan martial arts, some have made the mistake of believing the art to be one-dimensional, as we often see in modern Karate styles. Most people do not understand the rich heritage of the Okinawan martial arts. Some Okinawan masters fear that modernization of Karate and control of the arts by Japanese organizations will cause true Okinawan Karate to disappear in less than 10 years.

Several Kempo and Kobujutsu organizations have as their mission the preservation of ancient and traditional methods of Okinawan martial-arts training. In that regard, we must understand the two sides of the Okinawan martial-arts coin.

Many people regard Karate, the most recognized name for the Okinawan martial arts, as only a punch-and-kick art, focused primarily on striking with power. Others think of Karate as the art of the chop and expect to see a "Karate master" dispatch all opponents with the edge of the hand.

Actually, the many martial arts of Okinawa, whether Te, Karate, Kempo, or Kobudo/Kobujutsu, are full Uchite systems. As noted earlier, Uchi can be translated as "strike, hit, beat, slap, and punch." Those definitions indicate that the hand can take on many formations to execute varied weapons, ranging from the fist to claws, spear hands, knife hands, and so forth.

Yet the study of the Kempo hands is the study of concepts that extend beyond the range of the five animal hand formations and the way of striking common to Chinese pugilism.

James Masayoshi Mitose taught his Kosho Ryu Kempo using a pattern he called the octagon. This system was on his crest, the same one used by Choki Motobu. The crest contained the nine points of striking, which Mitose considered the main secret of Kempo. From these nine points, one could derive all the strikes of Kempo, as well as the defenses against them. The octagon became the source for developing skill and dexterity with the Uchite, allowing a student to train instinctively in the use of each skill by following the eight angles and the ninth strike, in formless patterns designed to create spontaneity.

The amazing thing about Mitose's Hakkakkei, or "octagon," was that he used it to teach everything in Kempo. Using the octagon, Mitose taught footwork, hand movement in strikes, targeting in Kyusho, and many other skills. He even used the Hakkakkei for a special form of training that allowed his students to develop defenses against other styles of martial arts. Mitose taught his students to watch movements and favored techniques of other styles. He then took students through the training process of the octagon and developed defenses against those techniques. This accomplished two goals. First, the students were always learning new techniques, "stealing" them from other styles. Mitose learned this concept from Kempo and Ninjutsu master Seiko Fujita. Second, Mitose's Kempo students learned how to counter anything they might run into from other styles.

Hakkakkei was regarded as the secret of Mitose's Kosho Ryu Kempo. According to Mitose, this was the greatest hidden secret of his Japanese Kempo masters. In regard to Uchite, which would have been the striking-hand techniques he learned from his Okinawan Kempo master, Choki Motobu, he followed the concept he had learned about the octagon. He took each of the Uchite techniques and worked them through the octagon, mastering the striking methods of Motobu's Kempo, adding them to the Japanese Kempo, and creating an unbeatable array of skills.

The Uchite were designed to cover every angle a person might face in actual combat, allowing the Kempoka to direct blows into the vital points of an opponent, regardless of the opponent's stance or position—standing tall, crouched in a wrestling stance, or lying on the ground.

In real self-defense, Kempoka understood that they never knew what they would face. Thus they trained to deal with any situation within the 360 degrees of the three-dimensional world. This was the reality of the Hakkakkei and the Uchite training of Kempo for self-defense.

TORITE: THROWING, GRAPPLING

Torite, one of the most advanced and important skills in the Okinawan martial-arts repertoire, means "the taking hand." Torite is the study of throwing from the Okinawan perspective. It blends the best of Japanese Jujutsu, Chinese Chin na, and Okinawan Uchite into an unstoppable skill.

Since the Okinawan martial arts began to leave the island, Torite has become the main "hidden" skill. The Okinawan royalty learned many skills over the years, realizing that it was not enough to know how to strike an opponent. In their position as peacekeepers of the island, they needed to be able to control and immobilize people in order to apprehend them and, if necessary, incarcerate them.

The Okinawan royalty built their skills on the Minamoto Bujutsu, which entered their island during the 12th century. Over the years, they added the Chin na, which came from China. But the Okinawans were themselves martial-arts geniuses. They improved on the skills they had learned from these sources to create an inexorable method of grappling that contained the special power-generation techniques of Okinawan Uchite, or striking skills.

In real combat, one never knows what he or she will face. The Okinawan masters understood that when they attempted to apprehend someone, they would need to be able to neutralize everything an attacker might try. Beginners learned to use strikes to weaken opponents so that they could use grappling skills to restrain them.

Intermediate martial artists were taught that they could go directly into their grappling skills. Should they run into trouble, however, they could use strikes to break the defense of an opponent. Later, they could return to grappling skills to immobilize the adversary.

Finally, advanced practitioners could go directly into grappling techniques to handle even an experienced opponent easily.

It is believed that James Masayoshi Mitose learned many of his advanced throwing skills from Choki Motobu. It seems that many Jujutsu practitioners did not recognize the sophistication of Mitose's throwing skills. They considered his Jujutsu mediocre, not realizing that he was performing advanced Okinawan Torite, a skill beyond their comprehension.

ODORI TE: MENTAL AND SPIRITUAL DEVELOPMENT

One of the secret skills developed on Okinawa is the practice of Odori Te. Legends abound concerning the development of this form of practice, but it is believed to have originated from the Minamoto Bujutsu, which Tametomo brought to Okinawa in the 16th century.

In Japan, where Minamoto Bujutsu developed into Daito Ryu Aikijujutsu, an ancient method of practice was known as Aiki Inyo Odori. This method of training combined several elements: special movements based on the harmony of energy, special breathing techniques and footwork based on the idea of negative and positive flow, and a concept of freestyle movement that looked like a dance but was actually a Kata, a form of martial-arts practice. This method of training is sometimes called simply Aiki Odori.

Because the same idea developed among the royal families on Okinawa but is missing from the Karate systems that developed primarily from Chinese sources, it is almost a surety that Odori Te derives from the same source as Aiki Inyo Odori.

The essence of Odori Te is in relaxed movements that are the focus of Ki. Odori Te looks much like Aikido but has a more deadly aspect to its movements, as seen in Aikijujutsu. Some people have incorrectly considered Odori Te as a form of grappling only, but the truth is that Odori Te contains Uchite as well as Torite.

Torite can be thought of as the grappling skills of the Okinawan martial arts and Uchite as the striking skills, but the process of developing them to an effective, even devastating, level is Odori Te.

Odori Te, as the ultimate principle of Okinawan martial arts, embraces not only physical training but also mental and spiritual development. In Odori Te, the idea is to concentrate the mind on each movement so that the body moves through the "dance" with total spatial awareness. The mind determines, with total confidence, where the body will be in space and time. Developing the concentration to move the body without excess tension takes considerable practice. The ultimate aspect of Odori is the achievement of divine inspiration. The idea is that the martial arts should bring one into harmony with the universe so that the source of everything—the creator, the Void (God)—becomes the heart of the warrior and the source of technique.

In the Orient, the concept of Kami Waza, or divine techniques, is accepted. This idea has not transferred well to the Western world because it clashes with the Western philosophy that the body is evil and the soul is good.

But in the Eastern concept, all of creation is good. The choices that people make are what determine good and evil. Therefore, physical techniques can be inspired by the Divine if the heart of the practitioner is pure. The Oriental world has always emphasized the heart of the martial artist. The idea is that if the heart of a warrior is not right, then the practice of ten thousand techniques will be worthless. But if the heart is right, then the skills will be right. It is said in the Western world that practice makes perfect, but the idea in Kempo is that practice with a pure heart makes perfect.

As the heart becomes pure, movements become gentler. This is the essence of Odori Te. The movements of a master of Odori Te possess a smooth, dancelike quality, light and without power. In truth, the emphasis is not on physical power but on mind and spirit.

In the use of the mind, the essential point is Mushin, literally "no mind," and Senshin, "mainly mind." Mushin gives to the Kempoka openness of mind and allows total spontaneity and creativity. Thus Odori Te has no prearranged Kata. This form of training goes back to ancient times, when the Okinawans expected to use their skills in life-and-death combat.

With Mushin, the mind is open and clear, ready to process divine inspiration into physical movement. The mind has no thought. Instead, it reflects like a mirror, seeing what is truly before it, with no preconceived idea of what comes next. In this way, the Kempoka deals with what is, not what he or she thinks will be.

Mushin allows the master practitioner to blend perfectly with the movements of one attacker, or many attackers. This talent is indispensable to a master martial artist, especially one striving for actual self-defense capability.

Just as Mushin allows the necessary creativity and spontaneity in combat, Senshin allows the power. In all the Orient, no martial artists are better known for their power than the Okinawans. Yet most people do not understand that their power comes not from their bodies—many of the most powerful Okinawan masters were small men—but from their minds and their relation to the spirit.

Senshin, which we noted earlier, means "mainly mind," and refers to undivided attention, singleness of purpose. We can best understand it as concentration. When a Kempoka focuses the mind on going from one point to the next, he or she uses a level of concentration that does not consider the possibility that anything could stop the movement. This is the idea of practicing Tameshiwari, or "test breaking." The student looks at the board or tile that is to be broken, Senshin concentrates on going through it to a point beyond the barrier, and then moves. The hand breaks the board or tile on its way to the point of focus.

If the mind is properly concentrated, the hand, fist, or foot will pass easily through the object. But if the mind is not concentrated, the technique will fail, possibly resulting in damage to the person's hand, fist, or foot.

Tai is the body, Shin is the mind, and Ki is the spirit. The body is the aspect of humanity that interacts on the physical plane of existence. The spirit is the aspect of humanity that is of the higher plane. The mind is the connection between the two, between the body and the spirit. When the mind is open, Mushin, and concentrated, Senshin, then the spirit flows through the movements of the body to create real strength.

Odori Te practice offers this to the martial artist, but only when he or she performs it correctly, as a method of unity between the mind, the body, and the spirit. This, then, is the heart of Kempo, the Odori Te.

Keri:
The Kicks

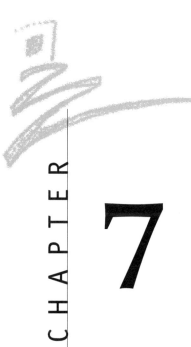

Kicks are the longest and strongest weapons of Kempo. It is possible for one to kick so well that an attacker can never get close enough to use the hands. But Kempoka must elevate all Kempo techniques to superior levels so that no matter what the situation, they can defend themselves. In keeping with the tradition of Choki Motobu and James Masayoshi Mitose, practitioners snap all kicks, retracting them faster than they are executed. Kicks travel circularly, up, down, or straight.

All styles of Kempo teach effective kicking, with some doing high kicks as a form of exercise, advocating only low kicks for self-defense. Other styles acknowledge the advantage of superior kickers in combat and thus teach the full range of kicking from head to toe. Flexibility, dexterity, and strategy are essential for effective kicking. One develops kicking technique, known as Keri Waza, only with understanding and experience.

It is humorous to note that some Kempo stylists state, "Kempo practitioners can't kick." Apparently, they have not carefully studied the rich history of Kempo from the Chinese and Okinawan heritage.

Northern Shorinji Kempo was particularly known for its full range of kicking. Okinawan master Zenryo Shimabuku journeyed to China to research the kicking skills of northern Shorinji Kempo, which he added to his Kempo and passed on to his students. He felt compelled to do this because his instructor, Chotoku Kyan, was the greatest kicker on Okinawa at the time. Kyan was the founder of the Shobayashi branch of Shorin Ryu. Many of the modern branches of Okinawan Karate originate from the teachings of Kyan. His influence reaches into some of the Kempo branches, as does that of Shimabuku, his student.

Much of the kicking in Kempo today comes from the great Okinawan master Choki Motobu, who taught James Masayoshi Mitose, the first person to teach Kempo to Americans. Kicking as taught in Kempo is always with a snap, except for the crescent and swing kicks. The lockout kicks seen in many types of Karate are regarded as a mistake in Kempo because an assailant can too easily grab and hold on to the kicking leg. This mistake originates in a mistranslation of two Japanese terms, Keage and Kekomi.

Keage means "kick up," and Kekomi translates "kick through." Some have taken Keage to mean "snap" and Kekomi to mean "thrust." With Keage considered a snap, the feeling then is that Kekomi must then be locked out. Taken correctly, Keage means to kick upward at a target above the location of the foot when it is loaded to kick, and Kekomi means to kick in a straight line off the hip. The Kempoka should snap both types of kicks, throwing the kick out and quickly bringing it back.

The practitioner must bring back all kicks faster than they go out, retracting the kicks rather than just relaxing the kicking muscles. Just as one extends a kick through tension of the quadriceps, he or she retracts it by tension of the biceps femoris. This technique protects the knee from damage caused by hyperextension.

Gaining proficiency with kicking technique requires a great deal of training. Kicks are such powerful weapons, however, that developing them is well worth the effort. Kicks can be three to six times more powerful than hand techniques and can be very versatile when one attains full flexibility.

KICKING SKILL

The three elements necessary for superior kicking skill are flexibility, dexterity, and strategy. Modern medicine has found a link between aging and flexibility, so people who develop full-range articulation in the hip and back will improve not only their kicks but also their health.

Flexibility

One develops flexibility through sustained stretching of the muscles. Thus a person should stretch moderately each day, working all the muscles of the body, particularly the hips and legs. Modern life, with its emphasis on sitting—in cars, at work, or at school—tends to cause excessive tightness in the legs.

Dexterity

After a person develops flexibility, he or she must attain a dexterity with the legs that matches that of the arms. Dexterity requires superior balance and muscular control. The best kind of practice is to kick at both normal speeds and in very slow motion. This method improves the manipulation of the muscles necessary to superior kicking.

The person who has achieved excellent control of kicks will be able to kick to the head with the same ease that an untrained person can punch with the fist to an opponent's head. Exceptional kickers can stand on one leg and comb the hair of another person with their toes.

Strategy

The next factor is strategy. Although many feel that kicks above the waist are not effective in self-defense, this is true only when one does not understand kicking strategy. Any skill used at the wrong time will fail. If you try to punch someone who knows what is coming, he or she will be able to counter the punch. If you try to throw someone prepared to resist a grappling technique, the throw will fail. Skills work only with proper application.

By applying proper strategy, one can deliver kicks effectively against an attacker's head or foot. Proper strategy begins by adhering to the principal precept of self-defense, "There is no first attack." Because throwing a kick requires a person to take a precarious position on one leg, attacking a prepared opponent with a kick in actual combat is extremely risky.

But when one has proper distancing from an assailant, kicks are excellent for intercepting the attacking movement. This is one of the principles for which Bruce Lee was famous, and around which he built his form of Kempo, Jeet Kune Do, the way of the intercepting fist. If an opponent is prepared for a high kick, then a low one will catch him or her unaware. If an attacker is prepared for a low kick, then a high one will land.

Ramon Lono Ancho (1928–)

A Hawaiian-born martial artist, Ancho had the privilege of studying under three of the greatest masters ever produced on the Hawaiian Islands. He began his training under Henry Seishiro Okazaki, the founder of Kodenkan Jujutsu. He then trained with James Masayoshi Mitose and William Chow.

A preeminent martial artist, Ancho found his skills indispensable to survival in the Vietnam War. Ancho contends that he would not be alive today were it not for proper instruction in the martial arts from his teachers.

Having learned Kempo and Jujutsu during a time of war, Ancho knows the martial arts as a form of self-defense and combat. Whereas many of today's martial artists are sportspersons and athletes, the reality of Ancho's Kempo and Jujutsu training has made him one of the leading masters of self-defense and true combat.

Surprise, the main element of self-defense, is especially important to kicks. Because most kicks require large movements, one must use them only when they are not expected. Moreover, a person who trains to kick in self-defense must work hard to reduce any telegraphing movement. With proper flexibility, one can eliminate such motions from many kicks.

Like hand techniques, kicks use both linear and circular movements. Many kicks extend primarily from the knee—to the front, side, and back. Other kicks use the circular swing of the leg from the hip. Some swing directly from the floor to the target, whereas others trace a circle in the air. Crescent kicks circle from the floor to strike a target on the opponent's head or body.

Most kicks useful for self-defense have a base leg on the ground. But other kicks are performed while lying on the ground or leaping in the air. It is possible to jump, spin, and slide in the execution of any of the basic kicks. Although these are difficult to apply in self-defense, one can sometimes use such skills.

The idea of leaping and spinning goes all the way back to the Shaolin temple. The idea was not necessarily to use leaping and spinning in combat, but to use it in training to develop strength and explosive energy in the legs. Today we know this as plyometric training, but in ancient Kempo it was referred to as Hichojutsu.

I will present here some kicks common to all Kempo styles, including snap kicks, thrust kicks, and crescent kicks. Described also are a few flying kicks, offering the reader the opportunity to develop strength and explosive energy through the ancient, traditional art of Hichojutsu.

Front Snap Kick	*Back Thrust Kick*
Front Thrust Kick	*Outer Crescent Kick*
Side Snap Kick	*Inner Crescent Kick*
Side Thrust Kick	*Leaping Front Snap Kick*
Back Kick	*Flying Side Kick*

FRONT SNAP KICK, MAE KEAGE GERI

You generally use the ball of the foot in this kick, although you may bring the heel into play too. The movement has an upward focus, allowing a kick to the stomach, a higher kick to strike the chin, or a lower kick to scoop up into the groin.

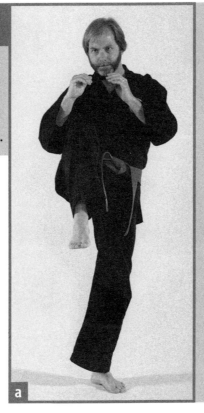
a

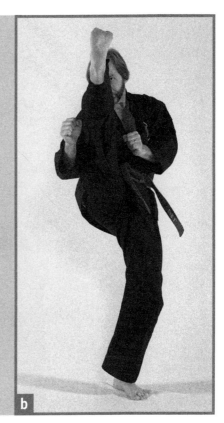
b

FRONT THRUST KICK, MAE KEKOMI GERI

Using the ball of the foot, or possibly the heel, you direct this kick straight forward, generally into the abdominal area. The kick can drive an opponent back, compress the stomach muscles to cause a loss of breath, or strike the bladder.

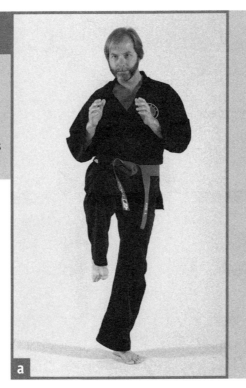
a

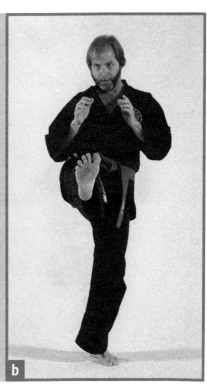
b

SIDE SNAP KICK, YOKO KEAGE GERI

For this technique, you use the Sokuto, or knife edge, of the foot, which begins below the little toe and goes back to the heel. Using this edge concentrates the force of the kick. You direct this kick, a Keage, upward into the throat, chin, or armpit.

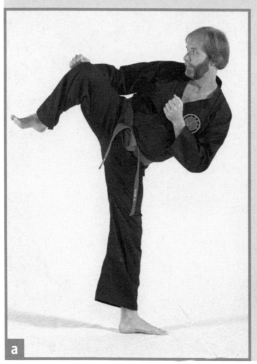

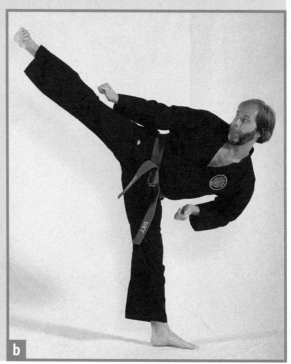

SIDE THRUST KICK, YOKO KEKOMI GERI

This kick also uses the knife edge. You direct it straight off the hips into the abdominal area and especially the ribs.

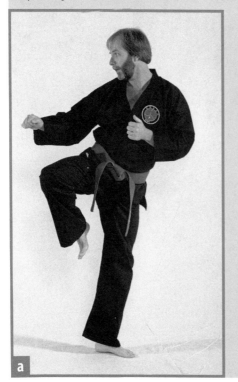

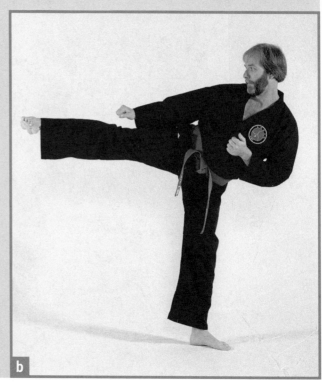

BACK KICK, USHIRO GERI

This kick comes up from the floor into a whipping strike. Although you can use it in other capacities, the favorite target is the groin of someone who has grabbed you from behind.

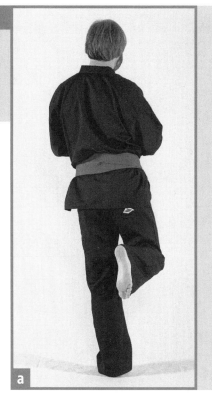

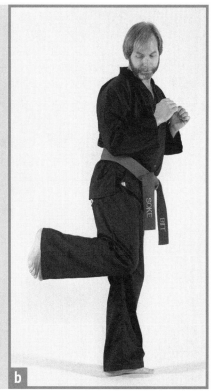

BACK THRUST KICK, USHIRO KEKOMI GERI

This powerful technique uses the heel as the striking surface. Its primary use in combat is against an attacker you perceive approaching from behind. You direct the kick straight back off the hip before the attacker gets too close.

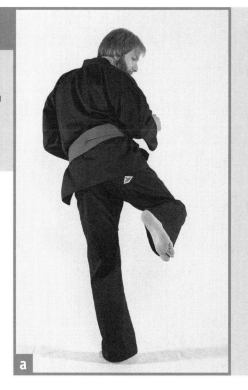

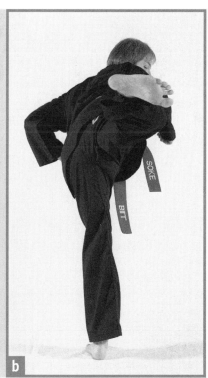

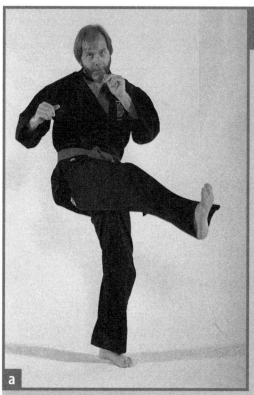

a

OUTER CRESCENT KICK, SOTO MIKAZUKI GERI

This kick uses the knife edge of the foot, hitting the target on the side by tracing a circle with the foot, clockwise with the right and counterclockwise with the left. This kick can deliver a heavy blow.

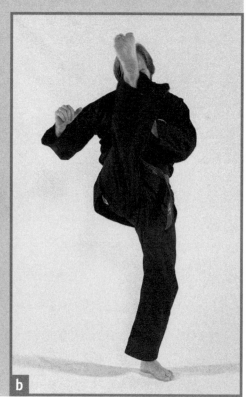

b

INNER CRESCENT KICK, UCHI MIKAZUKI GERI

This kick reverses the action of the previous kick, using the inner edge of the foot for the strike. You will usually turn all the way into a side position, bending the knee to prepare for a follow-up kick that might be necessary.

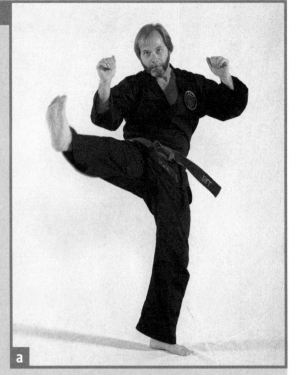

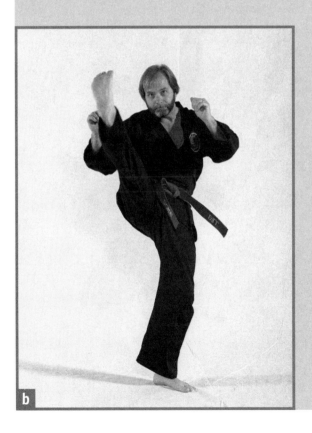

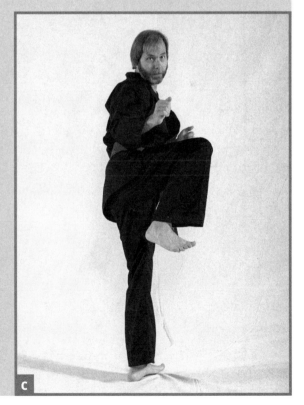

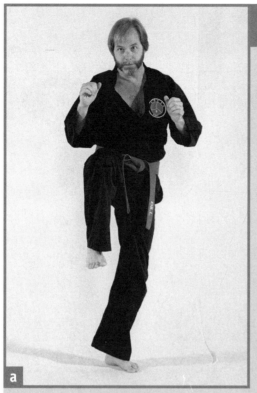

LEAPING FRONT SNAP KICK, TOBI MAE KEAGE GERI

This is a front snap kick that you perform while jumping into the air. The extra height guarantees that you can kick the face of an attacker, a kick that is especially effective when it strikes under the chin.

a

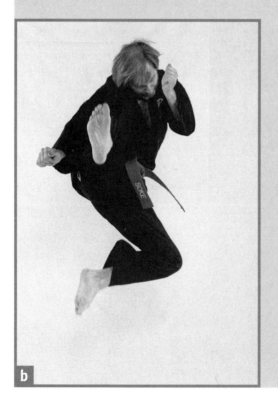

b

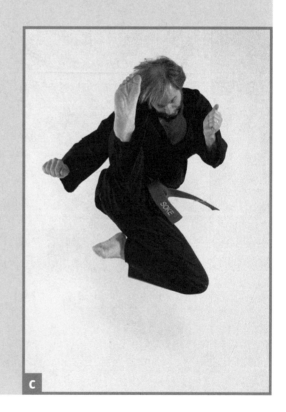

c

FLYING SIDE KICK, TOBI YOKO GERI

You can direct the flying side kick either straight or upward, with the force of your body flying behind it. Use it to strike a person in the face or, less often, the upper body.

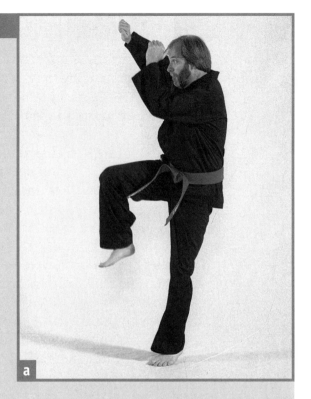

a

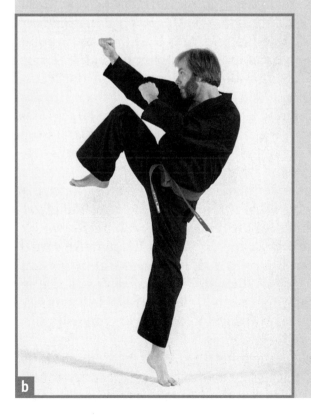

b

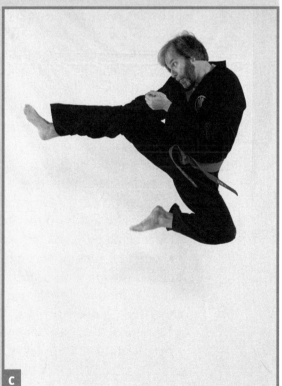

c

KERI WAZA: KICKING TECHNIQUES

Keri Waza means simply "kicking techniques." Most people must reach far for the understanding they need to develop kicking into a usable skill. Watch any beginning class of martial arts that teaches kicks. The first thing you will notice is how unnaturally the beginning students move.

Beginners make obvious mistakes in trying to kick. They assume unusual postures and seek to change their balance to accommodate their new skill. They throw their hands up or thrust them down, ostensibly for balance. Usually, however, these motions are attempts to coordinate the hands and body into the movement of kicking. The result is an unnatural motion that wastes energy and takes them no closer to the goal of throwing a usable technique.

Proper Kempo kicking technique requires one to follow some simple guidelines, the first of which is to move naturally. Mitose called kicking "foot punches." Although this seems ludicrous from the outside, when one compares it with the ancient Shizen Kempo, natural fist law, of Chinese martial arts, the truth of the statement becomes evident.

First, we must understand that Ken, from Kempo, means "fist." But in the ancient Chinese concept, fist is the accepted term for any personal weapon of the body. Ho, the "Po" of Kempo, means "natural law," as in following what is natural. When we consider that this idea was passed from the Chinese warrior monks to the Sohei and Yamabushi, warrior monks and mountain ascetics of Japan, we can understand that when the Kempo masters speak of kicking, they are speaking of natural use of the feet as weapons.

Next, look at the legs. In many respects they are simply like larger arms. They move in the same manner as the arms and have the same basic structure. How different, then, is the use of the legs from the use of the arms? The answer should be not at all.

Stand sideways and look in a mirror. Raise your leg and arm. Notice that they operate the same way, except that the hinge of the arm, the elbow, points backward, whereas the hinge of the leg, the knee, points forward.

This being so, you can use the foot as you do the fist. If you make sure to hit with the part of the foot that is a solid and effective weapon, you can develop powerful and efficient kicks. When you internalize this simple secret of Kempo, your practice of hand and arm techniques will help you understand how to use your legs. Then, as you develop your kicks, you will gain a better understanding of your hand techniques.

Some simple examples of this are the following: A rear hammer fist is the same as a front kick, a back fist to the side is the same as a lead-leg roundhouse kick, and a straightforward punch is the same as a back kick. To do the kicks naturally, we must do them with the same ease with which we move the arms. Sometimes we find that it works the other way around. A person who becomes proficient with a side kick may develop a jab that is more of a side punch, using the same movement in the arm that he or she uses in the leg with the side kick.

Remember that when you first learned to punch, you found it difficult to coordinate the hands and arms to accomplish those techniques. How much more difficult it is with the legs, which we use with less dexterity in everyday life.

The legs are powerful because they support our weight and carry us around in normal daily life. The more we are on our feet, the stronger our legs will be. A person who sits at a desk all day will have weaker legs than a person who stands on an assembly line, who in turn will have weaker legs than one who walks a mail route.

To use the legs effectively, one must develop dexterity of the legs that matches that of the arms. With proper training, this is possible, and with an understanding of human anatomy, the learning process, and brain structure, legs will gain the flexibility and adroitness of the arms.

When they first try to kick, many people immediately try to kick high, regardless of whether their muscles or balance are prepared for it. This unnatural movement will inevitably lead to failure and frustration.

You will often see people kicking with their arms out. The flailing of the arms is an attempt by an unbalanced person to keep from falling down. Look at a person punching. The legs are stable, or should be. The arms should also be stable when a person kicks. In the same way that a weak stance produces weak punching, so too do floppy arms give rise to feeble kicks.

When a person stands with the arms at the sides and then raises an arm to strike, the fist will follow an arc, moving from the extended position, to a bent-elbow position, to the point of hitting, and then back. A kick should follow this kind of natural movement.

Natural kicking is fluid. Many people, however, use a mechanical concept. They think of a kick as lifting from point A to point B, kicking out to target C, and marching back along the C-B-A track. But the leg must flow from one position to the next, capable of changing direction whenever necessary.

A good boxer watches an opponent move and waits for an open target at which to flick a punch. A good kicker must do the same. In kicking, however, one must raise the leg off the ground, so it is important that one can use a variety of kicks from the load position. Again, this is natural.

When a person holds the fists up, he or she has the option of throwing a straight-ahead punch, a back fist, a hook, or a rear hammer fist. In the same way, when a person raises the leg, he or she can throw a front kick, a hook kick, a roundhouse kick, or a back kick.

Working from the side-horse stance, the primary kick is the side kick. As the longest and strongest of all kicks, the side kick is excellent for self-defense. Developed properly, the side kick can be as fast as a jab and as hard as a rock. When one raises the leg from the side-horse position, he or she can convert the kick into a lead-leg roundhouse kick or hook kick without any telegraphing movement. Just as an upraised arm can execute many techniques, so too can the upraised leg. When the Kempoka has the ability to exercise several options, the attacker will be unable to foil the kick by adjusting to the movement.

It is essential that a kicker develop good balance. One achieves balance in two ways. The first is by improving flexibility, an important aspect that many people overlook. If the muscles are tight when one raises the leg to throw a kick, the higher the leg goes, the harder it is to maintain proper balance. The tightness of the legs can cause the person's body to become misaligned, resulting in a loss of balance.

Proper stretching allows a person to raise the leg and adjust the posture, so that the leg is ready to kick but not committed to a specific motion. Some martial artists raise the leg and must immediately kick because they have already lost their balance. If they do not kick right away, they will be unable to kick at all and can only put the leg down.

A good kicker should be able to raise the leg, pause, and then kick. The pause may induce the attacker to anticipate a particular kick, which may prove unfortunate if the defender can throw another. For example, suppose an attacker is moving toward a Kempoka and throwing jabs. The defender can step back to see if the attacker will stop or to ask the person to cease and desist. If the assailant continues forward, the Kempoka can then lift his or her leg. At this point, let us say that the aggressor continues with the attack and brings the lead arm into position to foil a side kick. The defender will simply whip the kick into a roundhouse or hook kick, which the attacker is not prepared to stop. On the other hand, if the attacker holds up the arms to protect against the roundhouse or hook kick, the defender can launch the side kick.

The second way to develop balance is to practice standing on one leg. You should do this in class and out. The more you practice, the better you will become. Start by holding a wall or by having a partner hold your hand. Then practice raising the leg and doing slow kicks in the air. Use your strength to keep yourself balanced but use the wall or your partner for support.

Then practice without support. Raise your leg and do slow kicks in the air without putting your leg down. Do a combination of a side kick, roundhouse kick, hook kick, front kick, and back kick. Then practice doing the series fast. At home, pick a target on the wall far enough away that you will not hit it. Raise your leg to point at the target and throw a combination of kicks. Always do both slow kicks and fast ones. To improve balance, the practice of slow kicks is best because it helps develop muscle control, which is the essence of balance.

When you stand on one leg, the muscles help focus the weight over the center of the base foot. The more muscle control, the better the balance. As you kick your leg out, all muscles of the body adjust to keep the weight centered. The more you practice, the more your body learns to make those adjustments. In real kicking for self-defense, you must instinctively make adjustments for balance. This comes only through repetitive practice.

Most important, the good kicker never does what the opponent anticipates. Some question whether high kicks work in real-life self-defense. If a person plans to use only head-high kicks in a fight, he or she will probably lose because the assailant will realize that only the head need be protected to foil the kicks of the victim. But if the aggressor realizes that the defender could land a kick anywhere on the body—a stomp on the foot, a kick in the ribs, a strike to the head—then the attacker will find it much more difficult to protect the body while moving in to attack.

Kicks are only the first line of defense. If the attacker realizes that beyond the feet are good hands, then effective elbows and knees, then grabs, throws, and chokes, there is a good chance the aggressor will decide that fighting is not such a good idea.

Too many people want to rely on kicks alone. Others do not want to take the time to develop good kicks. Both attitudes are faulty. At times, kicks are not appropriate. One should then use the hands, or grappling skills, or whatever. One needs good kicks; one needs good skills of all kinds. True Kempo is about excellence in the use of all the weapons of the body. But because the legs are the strongest and longest weapons, they form the first line of defense. The Kempoka should therefore be able to use them effectively. Occasionally, when kicks are appropriate, they are all one needs. The Kempoka who can use the legs and feet in the same manner as the arms and hands will have kicks that truly are Ashi Ken, "leg punches."

KICKING MASTERS

Among the masters with whom I have trained is Bill "Superfoot" Wallace, who has been called the greatest kicker in the world. Most people look at Wallace's kicking ability as an aberration that normal people cannot duplicate. Sadly, this is a mistaken idea, which Bill himself seeks to correct.

When Wallace developed his style of kicking, many considered it radical and unusual. When he practiced kicking by working freestyle Kata, people thought he had totally broken from tradition and was no longer doing real Karate. Yet the truth is that Wallace had rediscovered the original way of kicking developed and practiced by the Chinese and Okinawan practitioners of Kempo.

Wallace's lead-leg kicking idea dates back to the Shaolin temple, which had greatly influenced the kickers of Okinawa. History tells us that the northern Shaolin stylists favored the horse stance. This idea came to Okinawa, where it developed into the Naihanchi, the sideways fighting position of the Okinawan martial arts.

Naihanchi literally means "fighting inside a rice patty ridge." Because Okinawan martial artists might find themselves fighting on the ridge of a rice paddy, they adopted the horse stance of Shaolin Chuanfa to this potential. Many Okinawan masters became dynamic in fighting from the side position, with possibly the most famous being Choki Motobu.

Some people say that Okinawan masters never kicked above the waist, so that Wallace was again breaking with tradition when he kicked to the heads of his opponents. This is laughable when one considers the lives of three of the most famous kickers in Okinawan history. One was a tax collector named Takemura, circa 1879, celebrated not only for his kicking ability—the ease

Bill "Superfoot" Wallace (1945–)

During his early Judo training, Bill Wallace suffered an injury to his right leg. The damage was so severe that his knee could not stand the stress of grappling or even be used for kicking. Wallace, a dedicated martial artist and avid competitor, realized he would have to give up Judo and seek a new avenue in which to express himself competitively. He decided to try Karate.

Entering the Shorin Ryu Dojo, Wallace began training in the art of Karate, but when it came time to practice kicks, he could kick only with one leg, which seemed a severe disadvantage. The instructor, Michael Gneck, who had trained under Eizo Shimabuku of Okinawa, had his students perform a number of kicks with the right leg and then switch to the left leg. Bill couldn't perform the right kicks, so he did both sessions with his left leg. It turned out that the "disadvantage" of being limited to kicking with one leg was one of the best things that could have happened to Wallace. With that one leg, he developed a level of dexterity and agility superior to the other students.

Wallace watched some of the other competitors, studying what worked for them, especially in their kicking. He observed that some martial artists use primarily their front leg for kicking, without spinning, the way many stylists do. He also noted that kicks to the head could be effective when done with correct timing and strategy. He began developing his kicks, hoping to bring them to the highest level possible. Since he couldn't use his right leg, he tried to develop his left leg to do the work of both legs. The one problem he faced was how to hit an opponent on all three angles with just one leg. With two functioning legs, you can kick straight ahead with side kicks and front kicks, then use left roundhouse kicks to hit your opponent on the right side and right roundhouse kicks to hit on the left side. Since he could not use his right roundhouse kick, Wallace determined that he needed to fight with his left side forward at all times. This way, he could use side kicks exclusively to hit directly into an opponent, keeping his knee high to create a barrier of safety between him and his opponent. Next, he would use a lead leg roundhouse kick to hit his adversary on the right side, which was just perfect for his left leg. With all the training he had done on the one leg, Wallace's left-leg kick had become incredibly fast, allowing him to throw jab-like kicks with phenomenal speed. He eventually reached a point in his kicking where opponents knew exactly where he was going to kick but still couldn't block him.

But there was still the left side of the opponent to deal with. Wallace worked on throwing a hook kick with his left leg to strike the left side of a challenger. Once he had developed this kick, he could now hit effectively all three angles of an opponent with his left leg. He then began practicing strategies to get his kicks past an opponent's defenses. He learned to draw blocking arms out of position so that his kicks could sneak into target areas. He learned how to fool opponents into thinking he was going to throw a particular kick, and then throw another. In time, he developed the ability to chamber all three kicks the same, so that when he loaded a kick no one knew what was coming. Once he could do this, he ruled as a point champion, able to defeat challengers by scoring with his kicks. Most opponents never felt Wallace's hands, as the kicks were enough for most victories. Still, some people said that while Wallace's kicks were extremely fast, they were not powerful enough to be effective in a real fight. This was around the time when full-contact Karate was becoming popular in the United States. Full-contact Karate is similar to kickboxing but favors a Karate style of movement rather than boxing with kicks, as is done in the Thailand fighting art.

Wallace decided to try his hand at this form of fighting, wanting to prove that his kicks were real and effective. He proved himself by winning the initial full-contact Karate championship, becoming the first world middleweight full-contact Karate champion. He held the title for six years before retiring undefeated. During those years, Bill proved his naysayers wrong by knocking many of his opponents out with kicks to the head. His kicks to the body often sent opponents to the canvas, helpless and unable to stand.

Wallace's style of kicking was considered radical and unusual by many. When he practiced kicking by working freestyle kata, people thought he had broken totally from tradition and was no longer doing real Karate. But in truth Bill "Superfoot" Wallace had recovered the original way kicking was developed and practiced by the Chinese and Okinawan practitioners of Kempo.

with which he could kick the head was unsurpassed for his time—but also for a strange kick referred to as the scalping kick, which could strike a person at the crown of the head and literally split the scalp open, leaving the hair and a flap of skin shaking freely.

The next great master was Chotoku Kyan, 1870–1945, considered the founder of the first branch of Shorin Ryu. He was extremely proficient at kicking. Attacked once by a large crowd when his hands were full, he could do nothing but kick. He was able to defeat them all using only his kicks, which included blows to the body and head with his feet.

Finally, one of Kyan's students was Zenryo Shimabuku, 1904–1969. He so loved the kicking skills that he had learned from Kyan that he wanted to augment the curriculum for his personal use and that of his students. Thus, as noted earlier, he expanded the repertoire of kicks by studying northern Shorinji Kempo.

It has been said that Shimabuku was instrumental in expanding the kicking curriculum of the Okinawan Kempo Kai of his friend, and martial-arts contemporary, Shigeru Nakamura. Choki Motobu and Yasutsune Itosu, two of the greatest masters on Okinawa, had trained Nakamura. Motobu, as noted earlier, was a truly great kicker and excellent fighter. The mention of Motobu leads us to the last aspect of Bill Wallace's traditional kicking ability, his use of quick, snappy movements. People today tend to believe that they should lock out their kicks to generate maximum power. This shows a total misunderstanding of true kicking ability.

Locking the leg on a kick places undue stress on the knee, which can damage both the ligaments holding the knee together and the cartilage. The damage eventually causes severe pain in the joint and promotes arthritis and deterioration of the knee.

By snapping the leg when throwing a kick, one protects the knee and thus can keep kicking for many years. Bill Wallace throws all his kicks with a snap, retracting the kick as fast as, or even faster than, he throws it out. Many believed that this was not traditional, but study of the teachings of James Masayoshi Mitose and Choki Motobu reveals that this is exactly the way they taught kicking. The method dates back to the Kempo kicking of the old Okinawan masters.

Bill Wallace, from the need of adjusting so that he could kick with one leg, rediscovered the secrets of Kempo kicking—use of the lead leg in dexterous kicking, effective kicking to all levels, especially the head, and snapping the kicks rather than locking them. Thanks to Wallace, these methods have been proven in actual fighting and preserved for modern time.

Renzoku Ken:
Continuous Fist

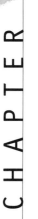

CHAPTER

8

What is unique in the practice of Kempo is the fluid combinations that epitomize mastery of the art. Renzoku Ken, which means "continuous strikes," is the self-defense method of Kempo. Renzoku Ken allows a Kempoka to deal successfully with an attacker, even one strong enough to stand up to a single blow. In Renzoku Ken, the practitioner reaches the highest levels of Kempo, performing combinations of kicks, punches, and strikes, which eventually can blend into throws, chokes, joint locks, and other grappling skills.

When James Masayoshi Mitose first started teaching Kempo in the United States, he primarily used a system of combinations to teach Kempo skills to his students. In the past, Kempo masters had spontaneously created combinations in their classes. Students practiced the combinations of the day and then forgot them as they practiced the next day's techniques. What the Kempo students were learning were the principles of creating combinations, rather than a rote series of movements. In this way, students developed the creativity and spontaneity necessary for actual self-defense and combat.

In Japan, these combinations were many times called Waza, meaning "techniques," whereas in Okinawa, they were often referred to as Renzoku Ken, which translates as the "continuous fist." Mitose himself called the practice of combinations Jitsute, literally meaning "real skill."

In English, most Kempo styles refer to the combinations simply as self-defense techniques. Regardless of how we refer to combination training, it is the unique and central aspect of practice used in Kempo. Although other arts use similar ideas, Kempo has made this form of practice fundamental to the mastery of self-defense.

Combination training has been termed the most dangerous aspect of Kempo training because it teaches the repetitive flow of techniques. Some modern forms of Kempo have preset combinations that link together 3 to 6 or even 10 blows. If a person gets in the habit of always performing such a series to its conclusion, it is possible that he or she could use excessive force. All forms of legitimate Kempo, therefore, have some form of moral training to prevent abuse of their skills.

All genuine forms of Kempo also teach students never to do more than necessary to end a confrontation. If an attacker launches an assault and a block by itself can end the attack, a Kempoka will only block. If a strike is necessary after the block, the Kempoka will use one, but only one. If an attack threatens the well-being or life of oneself or an innocent, however, the Kempo practitioner will do whatever is necessary.

In most styles of Kempo, the Renzoku Ken starts out very simply, mainly as a series of strikes or kicks. Sometimes Renzoku Ken are Encho, or extensions, of Kihon Kumite. This means that a Kempoka starts with a basic block, or a block and a strike, with which they are familiar. Then the practitioner adds one, two, or more movements to the Kihon Kumite to create a Renzoku Ken.

TYPES OF RENZOKU KEN

The two types of Renzoku Ken are the Kempo Jujutsu type and the Kempo Karate type. These archetypes actually blend into one in the advanced level of Kempo.

Kempo Jujutsu Renzoku Ken

Kempo Jujutsu Renzoku Ken follow the same pattern as most Jujutsu Waza. The defender begins with a block, performs some kind of strike that sets up a throw, joint lock, or choke, takes the person down with the appropriate grappling skill, and ends with either a strike or immobilization on the ground.

Note that the strikes preceding the grappling skill are designed specifically to make the throw, or whatever, easier to apply. For example, if a Kempoka blocks an attack and wants to throw the assailant backward, he or she might heel-palm strike the opponent's face, arching the assailant backward to make the throw easier to accomplish. On the other hand, if the Kempoka wants a throw to go forward, the strike might be to the stomach, bringing the opponent forward, thus making it easier to perform the throw.

Kempo Karate Renzoku Ken

Kempo Karate Renzoku Ken are usually a series of strikes. These combinations range from simple movements to complex integrated motions. These Renzoku Ken combine basic punches and kicks with animal methods and spinning actions. Each gesture can have multiple meanings. Applying these meanings requires Bunkai, or analyzation, exercised at every opportunity by the well-trained Kempoka. In most styles in America, these are the most common combinations practiced by Kempo practitioners. Because Kempo strives to develop effective self-defense skills, most of the Renzoku Ken combine truly dangerous methods such as finger jabs, claw rakes, and pressure-point strikes. For safety, most of the Kempo styles in the States follow the Okinawan concept of Sun Dome, which translates as "to stop one inch" (see chapter 2). Thus each of the blows are pulled just short of contact.

In this way, the Kempoka can correctly and safely develop the skills necessary for self-defense. People react in the way that they train. People who spend most of their time practicing how to score points safely in a light-contact tournament will perform in a similar way on the street. They probably will not have the skills necessary to defend themselves in real life.

But by practicing Renzoku Ken in a realistic fashion, a person will develop the kind of ability needed for self-defense. What is especially important is the targeting of vulnerable vital points. In sport martial arts, participants avoid the vital points for safety's sake, which is as it should be. But to become competent at self-defense, one must dedicate training time to realistic targeting of Kyusho.

TOITSU: UNITY

After many years of training under a capable teacher, one will have developed an understanding of the truly advanced principles of the martial arts. The most important of these is Toitsu, which refers to the unity of Kempo, that any given movement may be a block, strike, throw, joint lock, choke, or weapon manipulation.

Kempo Renzoku Ken here reaches its highest level, merging aspects of Karate and Jujutsu into one. Okinawan martial arts became the unifying melting pot of the Chinese and Japanese styles, resulting in this greatest of all understandings.

At it highest level, Kempo skills are all one. Strikes can also be blocks. Blocking movements can be strikes. More important, strikes and blocks can be throws, chokes, and joint locks. Kicks can be sweeps, reaps, and props, which one can combine with hand movements to create throws even more advanced. The accomplished Kempoka can also apply the leg movements of kicks in holds and joint locks, using them to immobilize an opponent in ground fighting.

BUSAN: CREATIVITY

The practitioner can also analyze throws, joint locks, and chokes to develop advanced angles and exceptional striking skills for combat in close quarters and against experienced foes. This is the heart of real Kempo. One learns this aspect by applying Bunkai to Renzoku Ken, which will bring about martial-arts creativity, known as Busan.

Without creativity, a person will be unable to meet all the needs of combat situations. When dealing with an inexperienced fighter, a lack of creativity will not be a handicap because basic techniques can easily deal with such an

So Doshin, or Michiomi Nakano (1911–1980)

Michiomi Nakano was born with health problems that seemed to dictate that he would live a short life. Thus when Japan needed a spy to go into China before World War II, they found a likely candidate in Nakano.

Sent to inform clandestinely on China's military movements, Nakano became friends with members of several secret societies in China. These friendships led him to begin martial-arts training under a Northern Shaolinssu Chuanfa master named Wen Lao-shi.

Nakano had trained in Jujutsu with his grandfather before going to China, and he trained in a Daito Ryu Aikijujutsu Dojo for a short time after returning to Japan. Around 1946, So Doshin founded the Nippon Shorinji Kempo system, which combined Aikijujutsu and Jujutsu with the fist-palm Shaolinssu Chuanfa he had learned in China.

assailant. But when facing an attack by a person with fighting experience or well-trained ability, basic skills will be insufficient.

Unscrupulous fighters who have developed expertise can be extremely dangerous because they have developed their fighting skill by preying on the weak and innocent. These criminally minded people have little regard for other human beings and no reverence for human life.

To develop the skills necessary for dealing with this type of attacker, a Kempoka must spend a great deal of time training in Renzoku Ken. By developing creativity in response, along with the ability to respond without thought, known as Mushin, literally "no mind," a martial artist will have the spontaneity to deal with any attacker.

By supplementing Renzoku Ken training, the fundamental building block of self-defense skill, with the other forms of preparation, the Kempoka can become a true expert in self-defense. This is the real goal of Kempo training. By learning to combine techniques, the Kempoka develops the skills necessary to excel in actual combat.

RYUKI: ENERGY FLOW

The final aspect of Renzoku Ken is Ryuki, which means "the flow of energy." All true martial arts emphasize Ki, the inner spirit and intrinsic energy of living beings. Ryuki is manifested in Kempo in two ways.

Aiki: Blending

The first is simply blending with an attacker's energy, using it against the assailant. The Kempoka can either combine the person's forward movement with the natural line of intersecting force from the defender's strike or join with the attacker's energy and throw the person with one's strength and the force generated by the assault.

Ryuki: Constant Flow

The second aspect is Ryuki, which is the constant flow of energy created in a Renzoku Ken. A grave misunderstanding is that one delivers the preliminary movements of a combination with little power, with only the final blow of the series being strong enough to do real damage.

If this were true, the attacker would have too much opportunity to counter the defense technique. In truth, one delivers each blow in a Renzoku Ken with Ki, the intrinsic energy. With little movement or windup, a well-trained Kempoka can deliver a strike of great power.

Ki power is a combination of physical coordination, mental concentration, and harmony with intrinsic energy. When focused into a blow, Ki power is devastating. Each Renzoku Ken strike is a Ki-powered strike. Moreover, the strike becomes part of a continuous flow of energy. Like the tremendous, continuous force of the wind of a hurricane, this energy blows away everything in its path.

Ryuki Renzoku Ken is an inexorable flow of technique that overwhelms an attacker. To reach proficiency with Ryuki Renzoku Ken, one must practice a great deal in all forms of Kempo training, especially in Renzoku Ken, the key method of Kempo practice.

Reverse Punch Extension
Reverse Punch Throwing Concepts
Knife Hand Throwing Concepts
Roundhouse Kick Throwing Concepts
Knife Hand Extension
Roundhouse Kick Extension

REVERSE PUNCH EXTENSION

(a) Uke (left) and Tori take fighting stances. *(b)* Uke attacks with a lunging punch with the right hand as she steps forward toward Tori. Tori side steps to her left while parrying the strike with her left hand. *(c)* Tori counter punches with a right reverse punch to the floating ribs. *(d)* Using the rotation in the hips from the punch, Tori follows up with a low round kick to the knee with her right foot. She moves her hand back to a defensive position to check a possible back fist strike.

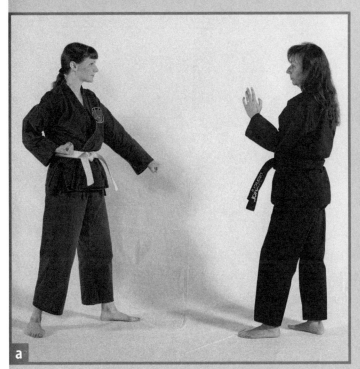

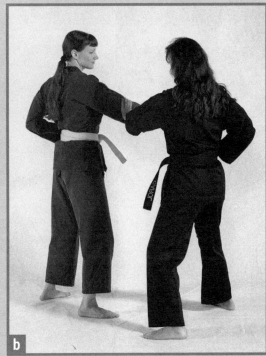

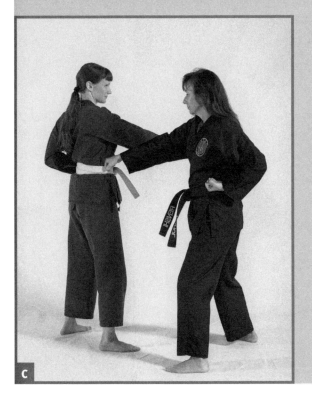

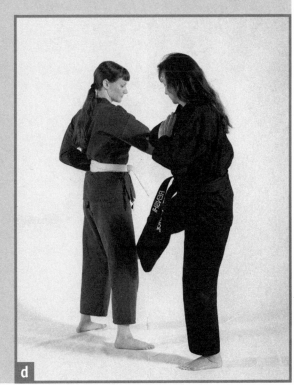

REVERSE PUNCH THROWING CONCEPTS

In the advanced concepts of Kempo, throws flow out of the movements as readily as strikes, as seen here. *(a)* The attacker begins with a lunge punch. The defender uses the flowing movements of the cross block, *(b)* reverse punch, and *(c)* roundhouse kick, this time to the head, which flows into *(d)* a strike to the head and sets up a throw.

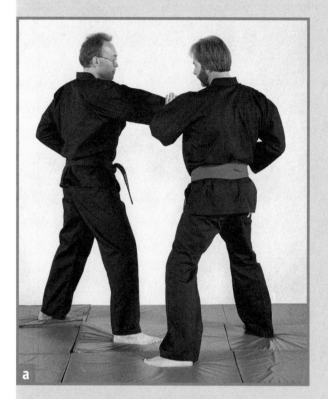

a

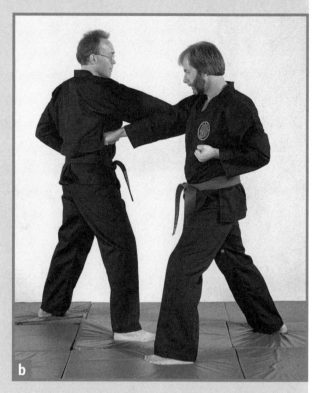

b

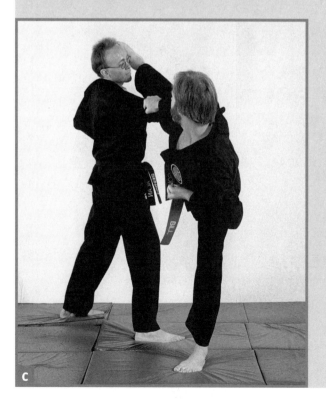

c

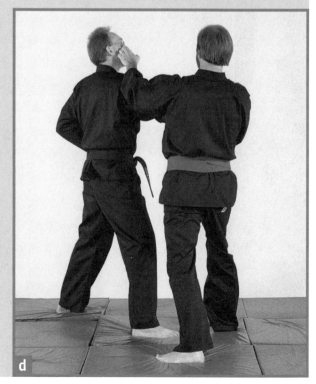

d

KNIFE HAND THROWING CONCEPTS

In another example of this advanced principle, *(a)* the attacker begins with a roundhouse punch. The defender uses an outer circular block to defend, which flows into *(b)* a chop to the neck, which in turn symmetrically blends into *(c)* a hook punch and flows back into *(d)* a head throw.

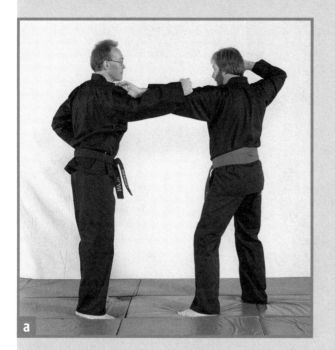

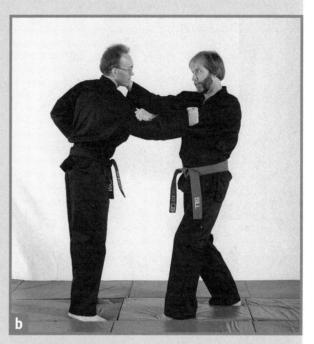

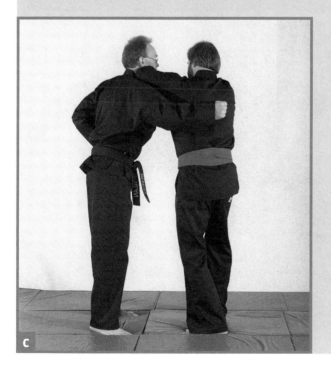

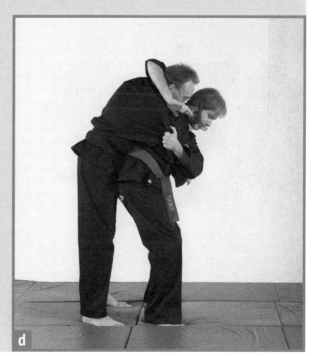

ROUNDHOUSE KICK THROWING CONCEPTS

In a kicking series, one can still move from striking to throwing. For example, the attacker begins with a back-fist attack. *(a)* The defender uses an outer circular block and explodes in with a roundhouse kick to the stomach. *(b)* He then brings the leg around in a hook kick to the back of the head. *(c-d)* As the defender retracts that kick, he sweeps it into the back of the opponent's knee, throwing him to the ground.

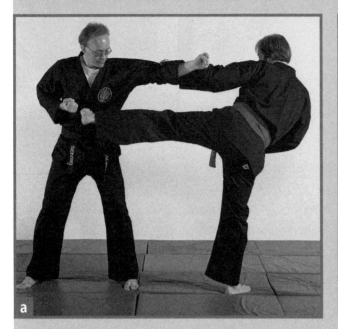

a

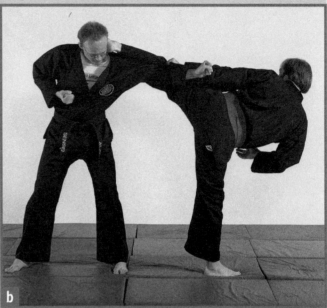

b

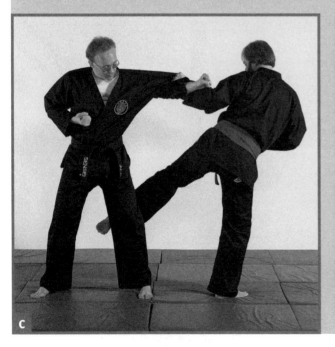

c

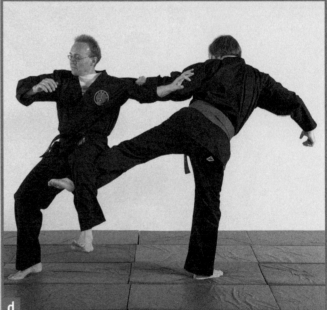

d

KNIFE HAND EXTENSION

In this example of Renzoku Ken, a striking series that one must master before moving on to the advanced skills, *(a)* the attacker begins with a roundhouse punch. *(b)* The defender blocks and counters with a chop. *(c)* The defender then performs a circular elbow, which flows into *(d)* a roundhouse punch, which then blends back into an uppercut.

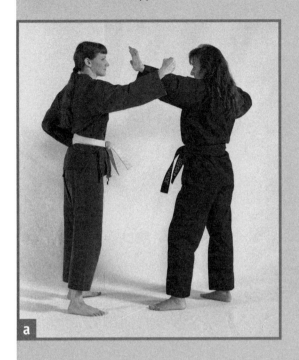

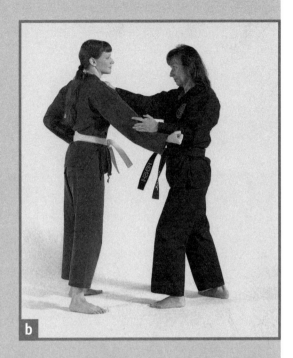

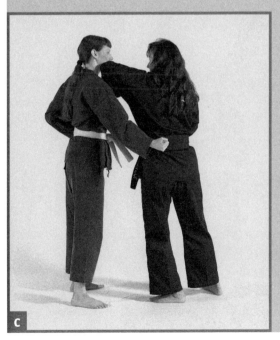

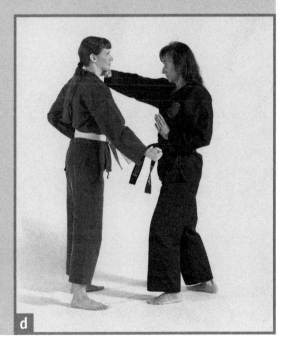

ROUNDHOUSE KICK EXTENSION

(a) Uke (left) attacks with a back fist to Tori's head. Tori steps backward to keep a safe distance between her and her attacker and executes a knife hand block as she moves. *(b)* After striking the wrist, Tori quickly grabs Uke's wrist uses as leverage while doing a fast round kick to Uke's floating ribs. *(c)* Without setting her leg back on the ground, Tori re-chambers her leg and fires a side kick to Uke's side while pulling her into the kick. *(d)* Planting her foot forward after the strike, Tori continues to hold her attacker's wrist to take away Uke's ability to block a follow up half punch to the same rib area of the first two strikes.

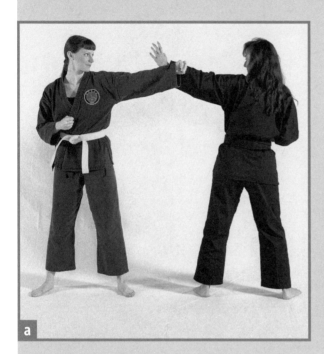

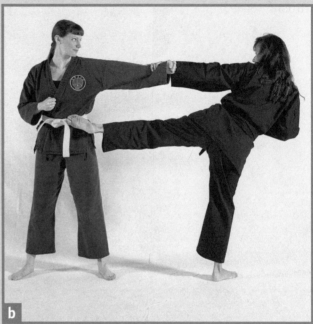

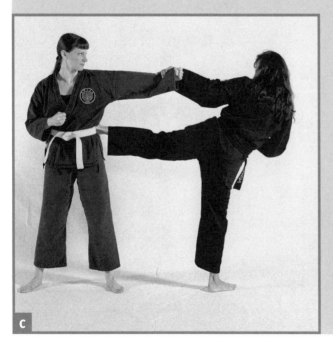

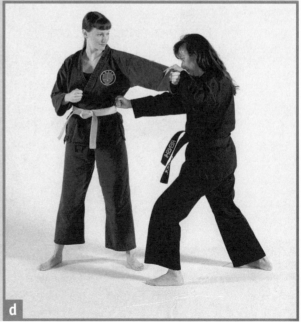

KEMPO PRINCIPALS

Two important principles of Kempo are Aite, the use of partners, and Kensei, awareness of symmetry.

Aite: Partners

Aite is one of the principles that permit safe martial-arts training. Aite can be translated as "opponent," but in the context of Kempo training, it is better translated as "partner." In this context, one must understand that a partner is someone you love and care about. When two Kempoka train, they are not trying to develop superiority over one another; instead, they help each other reach the highest levels possible.

Training with a partner has a significant advantage over practicing with a competitor. When you think you may have to face your opponent someday in a tournament or in a playoff to represent your Dojo in a contest, you will try to keep certain knowledge to yourself so that you will always be able to beat him or her. But when you train with a partner, you know that the idea is for both you and your partner to be able to defend yourselves on the street. You want both you and your partner to be the best each of you can be.

To withhold knowledge from your partner is to leave a potential opening in his or her defenses, possibly causing your partner to be unable to defend adequately in all circumstances. This is unacceptable in the ethics of Kempo. The goal of all training is to improve both partners. Therefore, as you train in Renzoku Ken and in all other forms of two-person Kempo practice, you should regard all those with whom you work as your partners.

With that in mind, you are responsible for the safety of your Aite. You must never do anything that could injure your partner. You must use each strike with controlled force, following the idea of Sun Dome to stop one inch from contact. You must perform all throws safely, using proper holding techniques so that your partner lands unharmed. When using chokes and joint locks, use the universal tap-out signal to keep the partner from unconsciousness or injury.

Martial artists can now participate in Karate competitions, Judo matches, and even Jujutsu bouts, but there has never been a Kempo contest and there never should be. Kempo is about peace and harmony. It is about learning to care about one's partner and his or her development as a martial artist. Kempoka who feel compelled to compete should find their fulfillment in these other methods.

When Kempoka reach their fullest level of maturity and spiritual development, they will no longer feel the need to compete against anyone. They will then strive simply to be the best they can be, while helping all Aite achieve their best as well.

Kinsei: Symmetry

An important principle of effective combat that one develops through Renzoku Ken is known as Kinsei, which means "symmetry." One should not underestimate this skill because it can be the difference between being better than an attacker and being unable to mount an effective defense.

The Kempoka should master three aspects of symmetry. The first, and most basic, is the symmetry between right and left. For example, if an attacker lunges at a Kempoka with a right-hand punch, the defender might move out to the left while blocking with the left hand. This means that the right hip rotates backward as the left shoulder pushes the blocking hand into position. If the defender then strikes with the left hand again, little power beyond the strength of the arm will be available because the body is already rotated forward. But if the Kempoka follows the natural movement of Kinsei and rotates the right hip forward, pushing the right shoulder forward and launching the right punch, the entire power of the body will be behind the punch. Then the Kempoka can rotate the left side forward again, hitting with the left fist, with the same force. Power is the gift of symmetry.

Kinsei is about using the rotation of the body to generate maximum power while smoothly and quickly shifting back and forth from the left side to the right side. But an experienced fighter might be able to anticipate this form of movement. Therefore, we consider the next aspect of symmetry—high to low.

For example, a defender might block a punch with the left hand and punch with the right fist. If the defender understands only the left-and-right aspect of symmetry, the attacker knows that a left-hand blow is coming and can be prepared to stop it. But if the Kempoka understands how to use high and low effectively, he or she can perform a counter that the attacker will be unprepared for. If the defender first punches high with the fist, he or she can use the same hand and a pivot around the elbow to transform that punch into a downward hammer fist that will strike the attacker in the groin. The attacker is unlikely to anticipate this movement. From there, the defender can shoot the arm back up so that the elbow catches the attacker, still waiting for the left arm to strike, under the chin.

Although these movements do not have the power of full-body rotation, they have the power of surprise. Any time a person receives a hit from a direction or in a way that the person did not anticipate, the effect is compounded. An old boxer's adage applies here: "It's the punch you don't see that knocks you out." One might also strike high and low using body rotation when it is evident that the attacker is not prepared to defend against such a movement. As always, Kempo techniques are a matter of doing the unexpected.

The final aspect of Kinsei is the symmetry of hands and feet. When possible, one should use kicks at long range, employing the concept of right and left or high and low. The art of kicking can be as deceptive as the art of using the hands.

But the Kempoka will also find it useful to use symmetry to switch back and forth between feet and hands to keep an attacker off balance. For example, the Kempoka can use a swift side kick to stop the momentum of an attacker moving in to strike. The defender can then step down into a punch, immediately shifting the balance back to one leg so that he or she can launch another kick, followed by another punch.

At its highest level, the idea of symmetry is to combine all aspects of right and left, high and low, hands and feet. When one masters this concept, an attacker will find it almost impossible to mount a counter once the defender gains the initiative.

When a Kempoka masters the principle of symmetry, Kinsei, he or she can gain incredible skill and ability in self-defense through Renzoku Ken.

Embu:
The Training

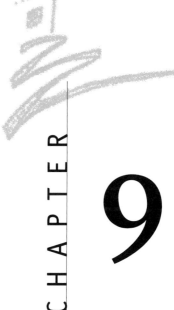

An important aspect of Kempo that has not transferred well into the Western world is Embu. In the West, students have a tendency to spar rather than train. Embu is training for combat, whereas sparring is training for competitive bouts. The controlled nature of Embu permits Kempoka to practice realistic skills in a safe way, thus preparing them accurately for self-defense combat. Embu includes many variations.

Special methods of practice that originated in the Shaolin temple were fundamental to martial-arts training. The two ways the monks practiced were known as Kata and Embu. We will deal with Kata in the next chapter and discuss Embu here. Embu are cooperative training sessions in which both martial artists seek to perfect their skills while helping their partners do the same. The term literally means "a performance of martial skill." Embu is commonly translated as "martial exercise."

During World War II, Michiomi Nakano, a Japanese man, was sent to China to act as a spy. While acting as a Chinese person who had been exiled from his home, he met the last headmaster of a Northern Shaolin branch of martial arts. That form of Shorinji Kempo was taught to him in its entirety because he was the only one interested in learning the ancient fist-palm art. It was such an archaic method that it did not include the five-animal style that most Chinese students wanted to learn.

After the war, Nakano returned to Japan and founded his own style of Nippon Shorinji Kempo and a new religious sect known as Kongo Zen. He adopted a new name, So Doshin, meaning he was the originator or headmaster of the way.

According to So Doshin, a special method of practice originated in the Shaolin temple that was fundamental to martial-arts training. It was known as Yen Wu, which in Japanese is pronounced Embu. This became the primary method of practice for So Doshin's Nippon Shorinji Kempo. Embu was extremely efficient in teaching the Kempoka how to apply their skills in actual combat while avoiding the contentiousness of sparring.

One of the mistakes that modern martial artists make is assuming that sparring is a traditional method of practice in the martial arts. It is unreasonable to believe that the pacifist monks who developed martial arts would have engaged in any form of actual fighting as a method of practice. Yet we know that the monks of Shaolin had combat skills second to none.

Monks, in particular, would have regarded injuring another human being, especially in the name of training or competition, as completely unacceptable. The monks would have needed methods of practice that allowed them to develop high levels of combat ability without contention, competition, or the possibility of injuring those with whom they trained.

Two ways of practicing Embu have developed in modern times. The first, the older method, has two partners moving spontaneously with no prearranged form at all. They move softly and slowly to maintain safety. As the practitioners develop their skills, they increase the speed. The targets are those of legitimate self-defense, the vital points.

The second method is for two Kempoka to choreograph a set of moves and practice it repeatedly. After they develop all the skills they can from a particular series, they create new moves and forget the old ones. These are known as Toitsu Embu and Goken Embu.

Regardless of which of the two methods one practices, the skills that one develops from this form of training are phenomenal. Embu allows a person to develop realistic skills in combat without having to contend against another person. In Embu, a form of courtesy begins the practice, which can be either the Gassho, the praying hands of Nippon Shorinji Kempo, or the Rei, the bow of most other forms of Kempo. One partner attacks, and the other practitioner blocks and counters. This goes back and forth. In some cases, the Kempoka use throws and joint locks in the series. In other Embu, after one partner applies a throw or joint lock, he or she takes the other down to the mat and applies a finishing strike or clearing technique.

In Kiyojute Ryu Kempo Bugei, students learns that a grappling skill should have the capacity to end the confrontation, either through a restraint hold, finishing strike, or unconsciousness-rendering choke. Thus practitioners generally perform the Embu as a give and take of striking skills until the Tori, literally "taker," the person being attacked, uses a throw, choke, or joint lock to put the partner, Uke, or "receiver," down.

The Tori can apply a finishing strike or a clear once the attacker is on the ground. A clear is a method of releasing an attacker but preventing him or her from being able to grab the defender once disengaged. One does this with a circular movement that pushes the attacker's arm away or slams the arm to the ground. One can also perform a clear with the foot. It is possible to use a strike-and-clear combination. Some styles use this method; others do not. As the Tori applies the clear, he or she backs up to create distance from the grounded Uke. This teaches the Kempoka that in real life a person on the ground is still a grave threat that one should keep at a safe distance. The Kempoka learns to maintain Zanshin, constant awareness, until the Embu ends. Thus in real life, as one backs away from a downed opponent, he or she still takes that person seriously. If it is necessary to allow the person to stand, the Kempoka is taught to be ready to defend in case the attacker renews an assault.

Although this book does not deal with the use of weapons, the reader should know that Kempoka also perform Embu with weapons. Kempo is primarily an empty-hand art, but some styles practice the full weaponry of Okinawan arts, and nearly all have some form of weapons training. The Kempoka must take extra care when practicing Embu with it weapons because working with the various implements carries with a heightened risk of injury. Kempo styles train with everything from wooden bludgeons and bladed weapons to flexible chains and rope devices.

Embu is considered an important form of training used in Kempo, second only to what is generally regarded in China, Japan, and Okinawa as the greatest method of practice, Kata. Embu is the predecessor of modern sparring. To traditional Kempoka, Embu is far superior to sparring because it does not encourage aggressiveness, yet it allows for more realistic self-defense training. Embu also teaches a greater sense of control and calmness, which are essential characteristics for self-defense.

Most of all, Embu teaches cooperation and sensitivity, along with a heightened sense of awareness. Sparring always has a level of danger, which keeps many people from participating in martial-arts training and causes many to stop training after a certain age. People of all ages can practice Embu because it is extremely safe, as long as aggressiveness and competition are kept out of the practice. In Kempo, Embu is an important and essential aspect of training.

IN YO: NEGATIVE AND POSITIVE

In all practice of Kempo, one must understand the concept of In Yo, negative and positive. In Yo is the pronunciation of the Chinese Yin Yang, which represent the diametric opposites of the phenomenal world, that is, the fundamental aspects of existence. As Chinese philosophy spread throughout the Oriental world, influencing thought and religion, these Taoist ideas helped people express many concepts, including martial-arts ideas.

It has been theorized that many Taoist concepts exist in Okinawan martial arts because the Taoist martial arts of Tai Chi, Pa Kua, and Hsing I, known in Okinawa under the heading of Ju no Kempo, influenced the growth of the Kempo and Karate that developed there. Thus certain ideas that helped the Okinawans express their martial-arts concepts would have been originated by the Taoist martial artists of China. We must remember, however, that Chinese Buddhists absorbed the same Taoist concepts into their teachings, so the Buddhist martial arts, such as Shaolin Chuanfa, Hung Chia, and other derivatives, would also have used many of the same terms.

ADVANCED KINSEI

In Embu, one of the most important lessons one learns is the concept of symmetry, a topic we discussed in the chapter on Renzoku Ken. But Embu offers a lesson on an advanced aspect of symmetry.

Kinsei, the symmetry noted in the chapter on Renzoku Ken, was about balance between the left and right sides, between the hands and the legs, between high and low. In Embu, the idea is to keep the hand, leg, and side of the body not being used in a state of readiness.

Shinite: The Active Hand

Symmetry is expressed in two different ways. First, the hand that one is using is referred to as the Shinite, the "active hand." The active hand might be blocking, striking, grabbing, whatever. When one hand is active (Yo), the other hand is passive (In). The passive hand is waiting, ready, yet relaxed. This is the Ikite, the "relaxed hand."

This concept is especially important in the striking art of Kempo. The Okinawans discovered early in their development of the martial arts that when one hand struck, it would do so with full power. It literally becomes a

Shite, a "hand of death." For that reason, the Okinawans usually strike with one hand at a time, whereas you will see that many Chinese strikes use both hands at once. Although the Okinawans include such strikes in their curriculum, which they received from their Chinese influences, they use them sparingly, and seldom in a life-and-death context.

The Okinawans avoid fighting if possible, but when their lives, or the lives of innocents, are at stake, they will fight with lethal ability. Even then, however, the Kempo stylist hopes to end the confrontation without resorting to a lethal strike. The historical record shows that when Okinawan stylists fought, they gave first aid to their opponents when possible once the battle was over.

Katsute: The Passive Hand

The passive hand was known as the Katsute, literally the "resuscitation hand," or sometimes as the Seite, the "living hand." This gave the Okinawan stylists the concept that although they might deal death on the one hand, they should be ready to save life on the other.

Seite has another meaning as well. When striking with one hand, martial artists tend to lose consciousness of what the other hand is doing. This ebbing of awareness causes a loss of Ki, or energy, in that limb. Should one need that hand, a momentary hesitation occurs as the hand is reenergized. In a true life-and-death struggle, that moment could mean the difference between living and dying. Thus the Kempo student is admonished to keep the waiting hand alive, ready for use.

Still, the advice to keep the hand relaxed, Ikite, is important. We know that a relaxed muscle moves much faster than a tense muscle. A strike, whether it be a punch or a kick, should be tensed only at the moment of contact, when the force is transferred to the target. Before and afterward, one should relax the muscles of the body. In this way, the speed with which one can deliver the strikes is maximized, as is the force. Always remember that Kempo follows the laws of physics. The rule here is simply that mass times speed equals force.

The relevant symmetry here is that each hand becomes the other in the course of movement. For example, in an Embu, let us say that a partner starts with a lunge punch. The defender blocks with the left hand, so it is the Shinite. The right hand is the Ikite, relaxed, alive, and ready to go. As the defender withdraws the block, the left hand becomes the Ikite while the right hand streaks forward, now the Shinite.

These concepts are not limited to the hands. Like all symmetrical ideas, they include the body. Thus if the defender performs a right-leg side kick, the right leg is the Shinite, and both hands and the left leg are Ikite. At least three weapons are waiting, relaxed and alive, to follow up the movement of the side kick if necessary. Add the other body weapons—the knees, elbows, hips, head, and so forth—and one has an arsenal, relaxed and waiting to follow up the Shinite. Thus the whole body is Ikite, relaxed and alive.

TOITSU EMBU, UNIFIED

The partners bow to each other to begin the Embu. The partner with the lower rank executes an attack, which the higher rank dodges or block. Then the second person strikes, and the first person defends and strikes. This process continues with the partners using whatever techniques they wish, aiming at legitimate Kyusho, or vital points. Whenever the senior rank wants the Embu to end, he or she simply says "Mate," which means "wait." Both Kempoka then assume natural stances and bow to each other.

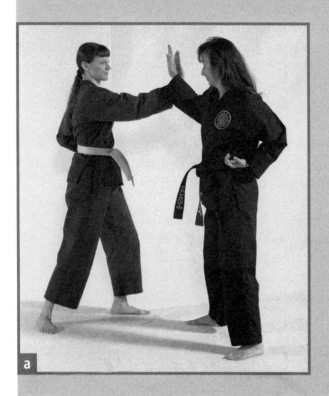

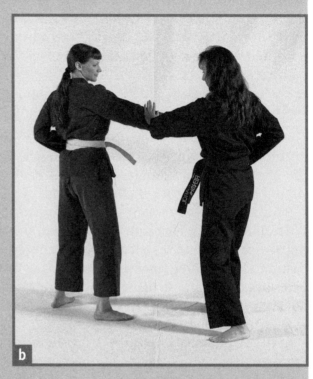

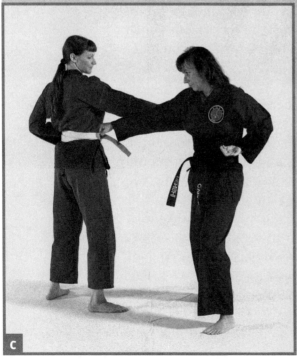

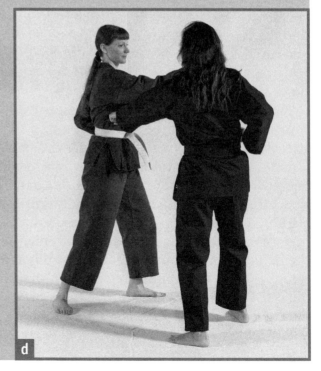

GOKEN EMBU, FIVE ANIMALS

(a) Uke (left) attacks with a mid-level punch to Tori on the right solar plexis. Tori responds by redirecting the incoming blow with a left counter grab and does a tiger claw strike to Uke's face. *(b)* Uke counters the attacking tiger claw by using an upward forearm block that allows him to set up his counterattack. *(c)* Uke throws a right reverse punch to the midsection while Tori initiates an inside sweeping crane block. *(d)* Tori continues the block directing Uke's attacking hand away from his body and strikes with a crane strike to the bridge of the nose.

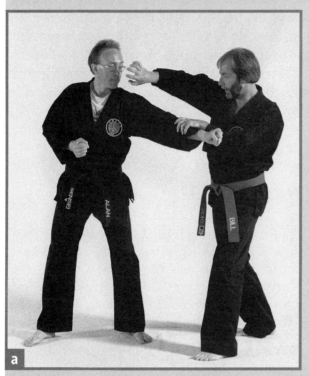

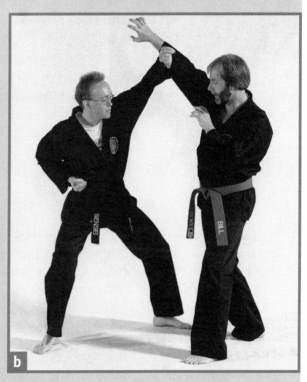

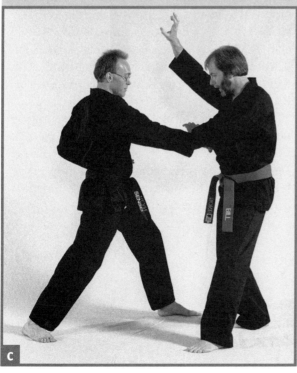

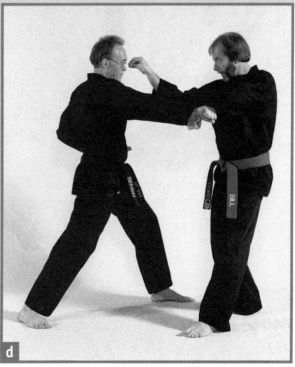

The great Kempo Karate master Gichin Funakoshi, the founder of Shotokan, emphasized the concept of In Yo. During his life, he was adamant that the Okinawan art be called Kempo Karate because of the philosophical meaning. Funakoshi realized that many of the expressions used to teach Okinawan Karate had come from the Chugoku (Chinese) Kempo styles. Thus he wanted the word Kempo always to be present so that the philosophy would not be lost. Funakoshi felt that if a person could not understand the relationship between the Ikite and the Shinite, he or she would never know enough about Kempo Karate. It was the idea of symmetry, of balance between the striking and the waiting, between life and death, that was the heart of the martial arts. Today, although Shotokan no longer uses the term Kempo Karate, others around the world have followed Funakoshi's wishes.

Bruce Lee (1940–1973)

The most famous martial artist in America is probably Bruce Lee. Years after his death, his books are best-sellers, as are those written about him. Lee began training under Yip Man in Wing Chun at age 13. He experimented with many other Chinese systems before coming to America.

In the United States, Lee began to teach a handful of students, primarily using Wing Chun. Among his students was Danny Inosanto, a black belt in Kempo under Ed Parker. Over the years, Parker and Lee discussed much about the martial arts and the limitations of many forms. After an encounter with another Chinese martial artist over whether he should be teaching non-Chinese, Lee began to realize the limitations of his original style.

Working with the principles of Kempo, which he had discussed with Parker, and with the assistance of Inosanto, Lee created a form of Kempo that he called Jeet Kune Do, "the way of the intercepting fist." Had Lee not been living in the United States, where innovation and creativity are admired, it is possible that he would not have developed Jeet Kune Do.

Lee used Wing Chun as his core martial art but adopted movements and techniques from nearly all martial arts, including boxing and wrestling. In true Kempo fashion, Lee included throws from Judo, locks from Jujutsu and Aikido, as well as advanced strikes of Karate and the animal hand techniques of Kempo, including various forms of Chinese Kempo.

Today, Jeet Kune Do has a following of people who teach either its concepts or tactics. In its comprehensive nature, Jeet Kune Do can be considered one of the Kempo systems to have been born in the rich martial-arts culture of the United States.

AIKITE: HARMONY HANDS

Embu ends with a throw, joint lock, or some type of takedown. The defender then hits or clears. This means that if the defender is holding the partner's arm, say from a wristlock takedown, he or she would hit a vital point on the partner's body. The defender would then sweep the arm away so that as he or she backs away, the partner could not try to grab and initiate some type of attack from the ground.

In performing a throw in which one is using both hands to grip, lock, or throw, the idea of In Yo, as in the use of Shinite and Ikite, has been superseded by another principle. This principle is known as the Aikite, the harmony hands.

Aikite is a concept that probably came to Okinawa along with the Minamoto Bujutsu of Japan in the 12th century. The basic premise is to use the hands in perfect coordination, along with the energy of the assailant, to blend into a throw, joint lock, choke, or other grappling movement. The Kempoka leads the energy of the opponent into a technique in which the person's energy brings about defeat.

The hands may occasionally work together, blending into a double strike, but this is an exception simply because the practitioner can focus more power into one hand than into two. The concentration of energy into one weapon produces a much more damaging blow.

Therefore, Aikite is considered mostly a grappling principle. Yet one must understand the advanced idea of harmonizing the energy of the attacker with the entire energy of one's own body.

Those who have witnessed the Torite, the grappling skills of Okinawan martial arts, realize that the throws and joint locks seem inexorable. Although they seem different from typical Jujutsu throwing and locking skills, their effectiveness is astonishing. This attribute comes from the Aikite. When the hands are moving in union, creating a vortex of energy, the techniques in that moment are almost irresistible. The great Aikido master Morihei Ueshiba used these techniques. When he began to move, an opponent found it impossible to break from his circle of motion or maintain balance beneath his Ki-filled hands.

Kempo throwing skills derive from the Minamoto Bujutsu as do the skills of Daito Ryu Aikijujutsu, which Aikido comes from. Advanced Kempo has more in common with Aikido than it does with modern sport Karate.

Most systems of modern Karate have become so immersed in competition that they have lost the aspect of Aikite and most truly advanced skills. Yet those arts of Kempo that derive from the lineage of Mitose have maintained, to some extent, a connection to the spirit of the original art.

In Kempo, the Aikite is part of the symmetry of In Yo in that it is the meeting point of the two hands when they are Shinite, in action, and Ikite, at rest. Aikite is the unifying principle that allows a Kempoka at rest to be fully prepared for an attack. Using Aikite, the Kempoka can unexpectedly transform blocking and striking skills into grappling skills. The hands move suddenly from being either Shinite or Ikite to blend together as Aikite to perform an irresistible throw.

United Hands

The hands can work together in three ways in Aikite. First, they can work in union to pull the person along a circular path into an inexorable throw. In this movement, both hands pull in the same direction. In a hip throw, for example, the left hand grips the arm of the attacker, the right hand holds the attacker by the belt, and both hands move to throw the attacker over the hips.

Circle Hands

The hands work together in a second way by forming a circle, with one hand pressing at one point while the other hand presses at another. In a typical Torite throw, the Kempoka uses one hand to press a spot on the lower spine and the other to press the head. This setup creates an internal pivot point within the opponent, causing him or her to fall. Many of the "floating throws" found in Aikido, Jujutsu, and Judo use this principle. The repertoire of a complete Kempo system includes all these throws.

Joined Hands

The hands work together in a third way when they join to create chokes. The hands can grip together in a forearm choke, or each can assume a place on one side of an opponent's neck and press toward each other. Finally, the hands can grip parts of the clothing with the idea of pulling together to create choking leverage.

As the Kempoka learns how to use the In Yo principle, he or she must also learn how to use the Aikite principle. When a Kempoka's hands, or more accurately, his or her body, can spontaneously move from Shinite to Ikite to Aikite, then the martial artist will possess an undeniable form of self-defense and combat.

Kata: The Ancient Form

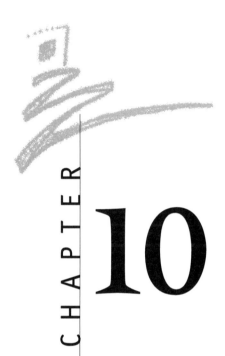

O ne of the most unusual aspects of martial-arts training is Kata, usually known in the West as forms. The shadowboxing of Western fighting arts resembles Kata. Yet the Oriental method of training possesses a greater depth that transcends the idea of boxing in the air. When performed correctly, Kata becomes the ultimate form of training, developing the human being physically, mentally, and spiritually.

In its most mundane sense, Kata is a mock battle in which the martial artist battles a group of imaginary opponents. The two basic methods of practicing Kata are referred to in Japanese as Yakusoku (prearranged) and Jiyu (free form). Yakusoku Kata, developed at different times in history according to the country of origin, are most commonly used today.

In China, prearranged forms were developed during the Ching dynasty (1644–1912) as a quick way of teaching a large number of students, people who opposed the corrupt Ching government and sought to restore the Ming. Prearranged forms were probably developed in the secular sector, with the monks continuing to use the original form of training, that is, freestyle training.

In Japan, prearranged Kata were developed during the Tokugawa era (1603–1868), when the warriors were no longer being called to battle. As peace emerged, the Samurai needed methods of training that would occupy their time yet not be open to abuse. Thus they developed prearranged Kata. Because combat no longer tested the mettle of a warrior, the learning and mastering of the forms became the test by which a person was judged. This method was preferable to the duels that some of the rougher warriors used to determine skill level. These duels ended in the serious injury or death of the loser. Later, mock battles using sport rules were developed, allowing people to compete in a relatively safe manner. Still, injury, disability, and death often resulted from these contests.

In Okinawa, because the martial arts were kept secret until modern times, the change to prearranged forms happened much later, receiving little emphasis before the 20th century. Sometime in 1906, the leading martial-arts teacher, Yasutsune Itosu, developed prearranged forms to use in teaching schoolchildren when the martial arts were adopted for physical education training. Among the warriors of Okinawa, the freestyle Kata remained secret, practiced only among the gentry. Eventually, the Japanese discovered the existence of the Okinawan martial arts and established rules and regulations for the "registering" of these "new" martial arts. One rule required an emphasis on prearranged Kata, the now-common method of teaching Japanese martial arts. In all three countries, however, some masters have maintained the tradition of teaching freestyle forms, which in Japanese may be called either Jiyu Kata or Mukei, translated respectively as "free form" or "no form." Examples of schools that emphasize freestyle Kata are Gu Lao Kuen in China, Tenshin Shoden Katori Shinto Ryu in Japan, and Motobu Ryu in Okinawa.

CONCEPTS OF KATA

Kata, whether practiced in the freestyle manner or as prearranged sets, are concerned with teaching the principles of combat.

Shingan: Visualization

First is the principle of visualization, which may be termed Shingan, although Shinzo and Shinsho may also be used. When practicing a Kata, the Kempoka imagines assailants surrounding him or her. The Kempoka then "sees" the attacks and moves to deal with them using Kempo skills.

In a prearranged Kata, the Kempoka uses prescribed moves, performing the same response each time he or she practices the Kata. In freestyle Kata, the Kempoka moves spontaneously, using whatever techniques will meet the situation. Both methods develop natural reaction, instinctive response, and the quality known in Japanese as Mushin.

Mushin: Concentration

Mushin has been called the most important mental attribute of a warrior. Literally meaning "no mind," it refers to the idea of moving skillfully without consciousness or self-consciousness.

In Mushin, the warrior does not have to remember what move to perform. The moves happen automatically, perfectly meeting the circumstance and situation. In developing this quality, those who practice freestyle Kata have an advantage because they learn the concept of spontaneous movement from the beginning. Prearranged Kata, however, can also develop this attribute if one practices for at least three years with proper visualization. Most believe that freestyle Kata develops the ability more quickly, which is why it was the main method of training for warriors and warrior monks of the past, who knew that they would see battle in short order.

Maai: Distancing

With proper visualization, which one develops by working with a partner and then taking those perceptions into forms practice, a Kempoka can learn many other factors when practicing Kata. One of the most important is Maai, which is distancing. A martial artist must work with a partner until he or she can visualize an attacker at the proper distance, at critical range. Then in Kata, where no real training partner is present, the Kempoka can practice realistic fighting techniques at the correct distance, with full speed, full power, and deadly focus. One must practice the Kata in this way to develop real combat actions.

Kime: Focus

Kime, or focus, actually translates as "decisiveness," which means that once a person commits a move to action, nothing can stop it. It is a matter of mental power, sometimes called *I* in Japanese, which means "willpower."

One can train Kime with a partner only by stopping the punch one inch from contact, to protect the partner from injury. If a Kempoka trains only in this way, he or she may develop the habit of stopping punches in a real altercation. But in Kata, against imaginary opponents, one can perform strikes with proper combat focus, one to two inches inside the body. This kind of power causes severe injury and is known in the Kempo arts as Naibu Hakai, "inner destruction."

Choshi and Hyoshi: Rhythm and Timing

Most Kempoka learn to perform Kata that have varying rhythms, Choshi. From this, they gain an understanding of timing, Hyoshi. In real life, people move at different speeds. A martial artist learns that by matching an attacker's rhythm, the attacker cannot touch him or her. By moving in harmony with the attacker, the Kempoka can lead the assailant into throws or joint locks or, by moving on the half beat, the Kempoka can hit the assailant. The ability to strike to a target at the right moment is known as timing. A martial artist who lacks proper rhythm and timing will receive hits from the opponent and be unable to hit effectively.

In Kata, the Kempoka moves with complete range of motion, from big circular movements to short, quick snapping ones, thus developing a superior level of fitness. Practiced at normal speeds for 20 minutes, Kata is an excellent aerobic activity.

One can also practice Kata slowly, with great deliberation, as a form of relaxation. In this manner, the Kata are excellent methods for combating hypertension. The emphasis on exact, precise movements will develop dexterity, agility, and a kinesthetic feel that improves the Kempoka's physical liveliness.

Through visualization, concentration, focus, and rhythm and timing, Kata helps improve a person's mental state. The greater acumen that a Kempoka can develop is useful in all facets of life—during the years of formal education, in one's vocation, and in family life.

Kempo trains the mind to be open, receptive, and focused, thereby improving learning, memory, and understanding, attributes beneficial in all stages of life. People who train in Kempo Kata from their youth generally maintain both physical and mental vigor well into maturity. Many Kempo practitioners live into their 80s or 90s.

From the Oriental point of view, the greatest benefit of Kata training is the spiritual dimension. In Oriental thought, each person has Ki, which we might think of as intrinsic energy, spirit, or even the individual soul. Universal Ki, which in Western terms is comparable to God, is the source of each person's individual Ki.

As a Kempoka performs Kata correctly, with a focus of mind that directs the internal energy, he or she becomes more aware of a spiritual existence. This awareness of personal Ki leads to a feeling of the source of that energy, which helps the Kempoka come to know the Universal Ki.

The beautiful aspect of this training is that it offers spiritual discipline without dogma or doctrine. Practitioners can take the enhanced spiritual

Rod Sacharnoski (1940–)

One of the leading masters of the martial arts in the world today, Sacharnoski began his training in Kodokan Judo at age 11. After entering the marines, he was stationed on Okinawa, where he trained in Isshin Ryu Karate, Goju Ryu Karate, and Okinawan Kempo.

After his military service, Sacharnoski continued to learn as much of the martial arts as he could, studying such systems as Dai Yoshin Ryu, Motobu Ha Shito Ryu, Kamishin Ryu, Shinyo Ryu, Shorin Ryu, and Seidokan. Although he practiced all the major martial arts, specializing in the throwing skills of Aikijujutsu and Toide (an Okinawan form of grappling), Sacharnoski always maintained the Kempo skills that he learned from his Okinawan Kempo master, Reisi Nakamura.

Kempo as taught by Sacharnoski is a complete martial art, just as it is taught in Okinawa. Kempo contains throws, joint locks, chokes, strikes, punches, kicks, and weapons training. Kempo as taught in Juko Kai focuses on self-defense, without a sporting aspect. It emphasizes powerful striking and kicking, along with devastating throws and locks, with a focus on practical application.

awareness and apply it as they wish, in whatever faith or denomination they choose to express their religious feelings. Even those without a particular religious inclination tend to find their spiritual focus through dedicated Kata training.

This facet of Kata practice has always been at the heart of classical Kempo training. Although not all Kempo schools emphasize it, those of a more traditional nature continue to admonish their students to seek spiritual enlightenment along with the many other benefits of Kempo.

Some modern Kempo styles refer to Kata training with other names. Some of the Chinese arts refer to each form as a Chuan or Kuen, which means "fist" but is used in reference to form practice. English-speaking Kempoka sometimes refer to Kata training as forms. Most styles with a Japanese or Okinawan influence use the word Kata. Nippon Shorinji Kempo, however, prefers not to use the word Kata, using instead the Japanese pronunciation of fist, Ken, or the formal designation, Hokei, method form, which have both single-person and two-person training routines.

Regardless of the name, some style of Kata training is essential for proper development of the martial artist. Innumerable masters, especially those of the Okinawan tradition, believe Kata to be the heart of Kempo. One should engage in Kata training daily. It develops the whole being—physical skills, mental discernment, and spiritual insight. A true Kempo instructor, of any level of knowledge, will stress the necessity of Kata training. Three of the Kata are presented here. The other three are Koken Kata, Sanchin Kata, and Taikyoku Kata.

Toitsu Kata

Goken Kata

Keri Kata

TOITSU KATA

(a) Like all Kata in the Kempo system you start the form with a bow to show respect to the innovators and decendents of the art. *(b)* Start by turning to the left to face an imaginary opponent and execute a knife hand strike with the left hand in high horse stance. The right hand moves at the same time to a position next to the right ear chambering it for the next move. *(c)* Now turn body completely to the left into a forward stance to execute a knife hand strike to your opponent's temple or jaw. *(d)* Snap the hips forward as you execute a left straight or reverse punch. Keep your weight balanced equally on both legs.

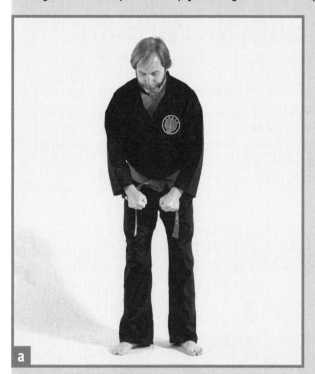

a

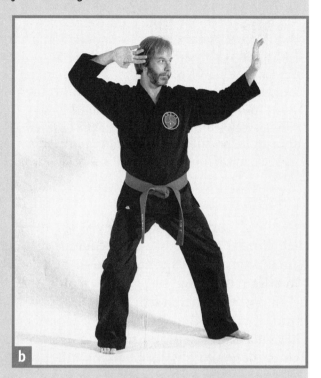

b

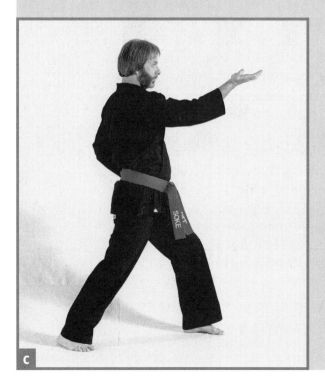

c

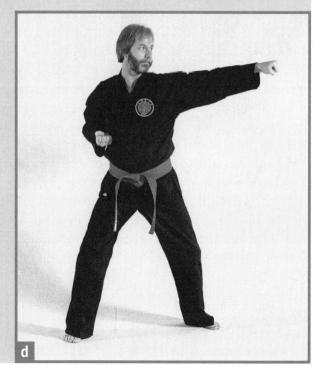

d

(e) Using the same hand you will do a back fist strike by quickly dropping your hand to your front hip at belt level and snapping the hand back to the attacker's head. *(f)* Quickly turn right to look for a possible second attacker for a moment.

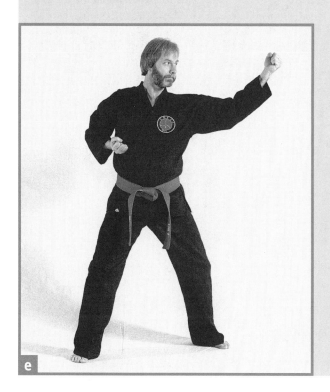

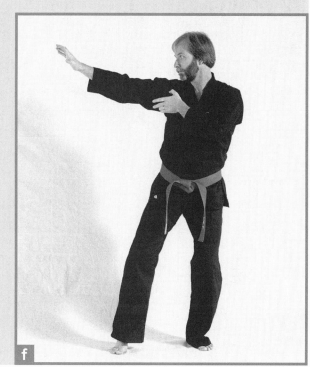

GOKEN KATA

(a) After bowing start the kata by moving to your left at a 45 degree angle. At the moment your foot stops moving into a horse stance do a high or overhead tiger claw block with the left hand and low tiger grab with the right hand. With the right hand you would concentrate on grabbing a spot under the floating ribs, your imaginary opponent's belt, or his clothing. *(b)* Pull the right hand back with a snapping motion to your body at the same time your left hand does a tiger claw to your opponent's head or chest. *(c)* Turn to the right 45 degree mark moving into a cat stance with the right foot forward. The hands move into the classical twin snakes coil to strike position. *(d)* With the right hand execute a snake strike to the eyes of your second imaginary opponent while remaining in a cat stance.

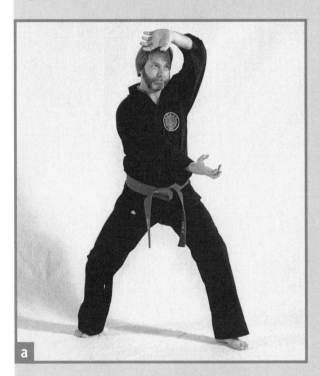

a

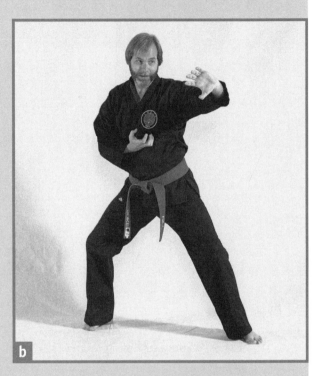

b

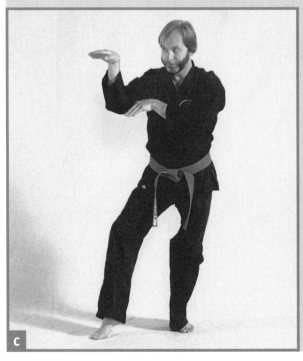

c

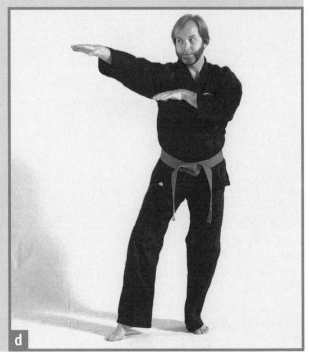

d

(e) Switching to a new animal, block your attacker's counter with a right inward crane block. *(f)* Circle the right hand downward to open up your target and use a crane strike to the throat or eyes. Finish the Kata with a bow.

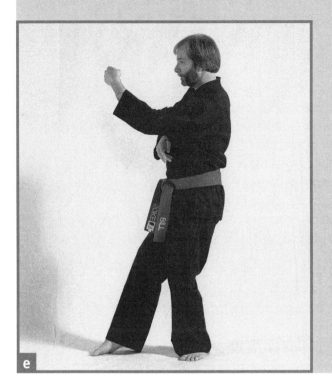

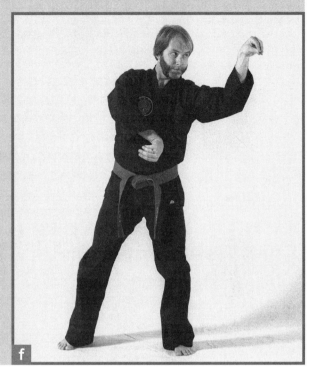

135

KERI KATA

Kicking is one of the most important skills of Kempo because it has the potential to keep an attacker at long range. You can direct kicks upward, downward, or straight off the hip. You can execute them forward, sideways, or backward, in inner or outer circles. You can use a kick to attack from every angle.

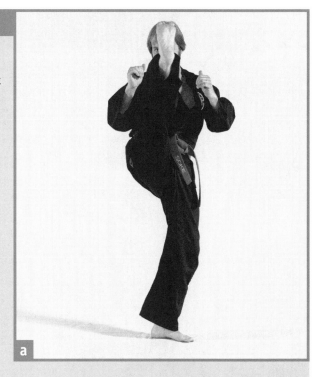

a

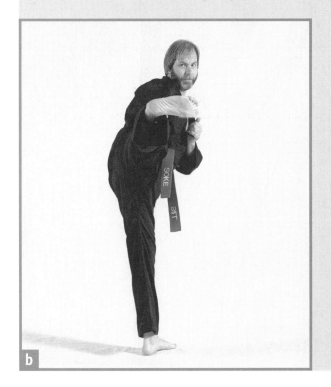

b

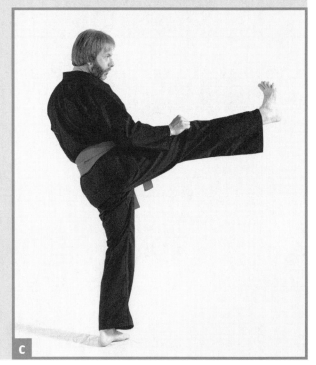

c

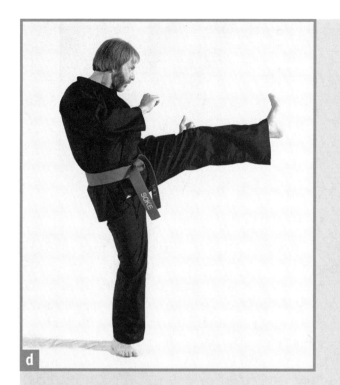

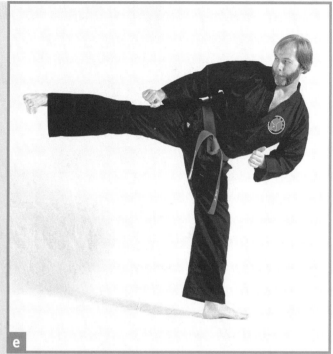

KERI KATA   *(continued)*

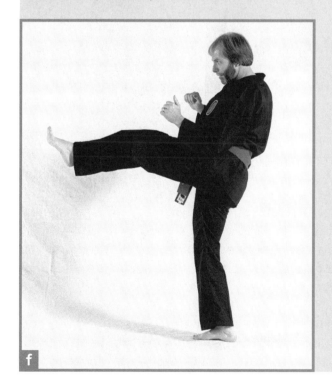

KEMPO NO RITSUDO TO NAGARE

Learning a memorized set of techniques, whether in the form of Kata or in the form of Waza (technique), violates the concepts of Kempo. In the methods of ancient Kempo, both Japanese and Okinawan, two principles, Ritsudo and Nagare Komi, summarize the concept of the effectiveness of the flow.

Ritsudo

Ritsudo is rhythmic movement founded in the concepts of Maai, distancing; Choshi, rhythm; and Hyoshi, timing.

Maai: Distancing

Distancing is a part of the rhythm of a fight. It is extremely important to maintain proper distance from an attacker. An attacker standing within striking distance can hit the defender before he or she has an opportunity to perform any kind of countermove, either a dodge or a block. Proper distancing gives the defender time to perceive an attack and react to it. Without sufficient time, one cannot defend properly. Ma, referring to interval, and Ai, referring to union, reflect the musical concept of rhythm. Each movement is a beat. The time required to reach from point A to point B constitutes the beat of a fight.

Choshi: Rhythm

Choshi is the rhythm that allows the defender to match an attacker's movement so that no matter how hard the attacker may try to hit the defender, the defender can stay just out of touch. Real fighting is moving in rhythm to make sure that an assailant's attacks miss while moving into position to strike. Bruce Lee called this "hitting on the half-beat."

Hyoshi: Timing

Learning to use sufficient time to close the gap allows the Kempoka to develop timing in a fight. This is Hyoshi. Timing is the ability to strike with a technique or capture the assailant's movement so that one can apply countermoves. It is possible to punch too fast or too slow. Obviously, a strike delivered too slowly will allow the opponent to move out of the way of the weapon. A strike delivered too quickly can occupy a space before the target reaches that spot. For example, let us say that you throw a right jab at a person's face. Each time, you notice that the person dodges the head to the left. So the next time you throw your punch, you aim to the spot where you know the person moves. If you punch too fast, however, your strike will arrive at the site before the attacker's head, and you will miss. If you watch boxing or full-contact Karate bouts, especially among amateurs, you will see this occur many times.

Thus Ritsudo, rhythmic movement in a fight, calls for the Kempoka to maintain proper distancing and thus have time to react to an attack. Next, one needs rhythm to avoid being hit by the attack. Finally, one needs timing to hit, throw, or joint lock the assailant or use other technique to subdue the attacker. Thus Ritsudo includes Maai, Choshi, and Hyoshi. This has been considered the secret of the ancient Okinawan martial art of Bushi Te and is usually referred to as Odorite, literally "the dancing hand."

Nagare Komi: Flow

The next aspect of the flow of Kempo is Nagare Komi, which literally means "to flow in." Nagare itself means the flow of anything—a river, the air, life, or combat. In the Oriental way of thinking, as it developed in Taoism and influenced Buddhism, all of life is a flow. To learn to move in harmony with the flow is to master living. In combat, to master the flow of the fight is to master the martial arts.

In Nagare Komi, the idea is that each motion—following the law of nature, the construction of the human body, and the concepts of physics as expressed in the laws of energy and motion— should naturally flow into the next movement. What in Kempo we commonly call techniques are examples of this flow. In the past, the masters demonstrated extemporaneously their understanding of flow and encouraged their students to practice until they could come into an intuitive understanding of this flow.

Thus the idea is that from one move to the next, there is a Nagare Komi, a flowing into. One must understand this flow in three dimensions. It is not enough to understand the existence of a flow; one must know how the flow affects target availability. Thus the Kempoka can use the flow in three basic manners.

Lateral Symmetry

First is lateral symmetry, which refers to striking left, right, left, and so on. This is easiest to see in hand techniques and in the use of the hip for power generation. As the right hand strikes, the left prepares to deliver the next strike with full hip rotation for power, and so on with the right hand again if necessary.

Vertical Symmetry

Next is vertical symmetry, harmony in the use of hands and legs. Just as a person flows easily from one hand to the next, he or she should flow with the legs and the hands. This type of symmetry usually involves lateral movement as well, depending on which targets are open to attack.

Single Symmetry

The third manner is single symmetry. This opportunity usually occurs with the hands, although now many people have the balance and dexterity to use their kicks in this fashion. Single symmetry refers to an opportunity to block with one hand and turn that block into a strike and possibly into a second.

Each of these cases must involve Nagare Komi, the flowing of each motion into the next with no waste of time and with time used in proper rhythm. Each strike thus lands on the most available target, achieving the maximum effect for an effective self-defense combination. For Nagare Komi to be effective, the Kempoka must master Ritsudo. An unfocused, off-target, and mistimed flow of techniques will be ineffective. For that reason, one who simply memorizes techniques will not be capable of effective self-defense. A person can know hundreds of Waza but not have an understanding of timing, rhythm, distancing, rhythmic movement, or flow.

It is time that Kempo practitioners, regardless of style, return to the basics of true martial-arts practice. They must research the facets of Ritsudo and Nagare Komi as preserved in the ancient forms of Kempo that make up the foundation of the Japanese and Okinawan Bujutsu. They must understand the Takeumu, martial creativity, of the Minamoto martial arts as preserved in the arts of Ueshiba's Aikido as well as the Odorite maintained in the ancient Okinawan Bujutsu. They must realize that it is not enough to memorize Waza or Kata, that instead they must have an intuitive understanding of the principles that are the foundation of those combinations. Most of all, they must comprehend the freedom of motion as taught in Jiyu (freestyle) methods of Kata and Embu, the ancient forms of practice. When Kempo practitioners attain these understandings, then they will know the flow of Kempo.

KI

The essence of all martial-arts training is found in the concept of Ki, the essential energy that created the universe. This is a concept that developed in Taoist philosophy and has been absorbed into nearly every aspect of Oriental life, including the martial arts. All true martial arts systems are Kijutsu, or "spirit arts."

Ki can be translated as "spirit," "energy," "intrinsic energy," and "air." It has even more meanings, which lend themselves to the attitude and nature of man, such as "mood," "intention," "temper," and "essence," all relating to the heart or soul of being. Ki literally has the tendency to be everything, the foundation of life at its most profound level.

All higher-level abilities of the martial arts are attributed to Ki, so, of course, Ki is one of the most important aspects of Kata development. If Kata did not have the potential to improve the flow and development of Ki, it would not be part of martial-arts training.

Kata training can be the most spiritual aspect of practice. First, before going into the more esoteric aspect of Kata Ki training, we will look at the three forms of Ki essential to Kata practice.

Kiai: Spiritual Harmony

The first is Kiai, which translates as "spiritual harmony." On a more mundane level, it can mean "energy united." This refers to the ability of a Kempoka to focus all physical and mental energy into one point, say the two knuckles of the forefist. A 120-pound person who can concentrate all of his or her body power into a punch can easily produce the 20 pounds of pressure sufficient to break particular bones or damage certain organs. The ability to draw on the full power of one's united energy is a great attribute indeed for self-defense.

Kiai requires the harmony of body mechanics with the total focus of the mind. This convergence is called Kime. One learns this aspect by training to look where one is punching and training the body to strike where it is looking. This teaches the union of mind and body, many times referred to as Shin Shin, literally "mind and body."

Yet to maximize the totality of the mind and body union is to introduce into it the aspect of spirit. This is the Ki. One accomplishes it by coordinating the breath, Ibuki, with the movement. To achieve maximum power, the outer breath must occur at the point of striking. Instructors of many Kempo, Karate, and Kobujutsu styles encourage their students to yell at the moment of hitting. The yell insures that the person is breathing out at the same time he or she is making the hit.

Of course, it is not the yell that is important; it is the breathing out. By breathing out as one strikes, the person focuses not only the body and mind into the strike but also the spirit, the Ki. When one performs a Ki strike, he or she feels the energy inside the body, not just on the outside.

From a self-defense point of view, this means that small people can stop bigger people because they hit not with only with their bodies and minds but also with their inner strength, their spirit. This, the Orientals believe, is the greatest of all power.

Kiai teaches the lesson of concentration. The application to daily living is that people should concentrate only on what they are doing at the time they are doing it. Consider the child who is thinking of playing when he or she is doing homework. The child will do the homework poorly and will receive mediocre grades. Moreover, the child who is aware that he or she is doing inferior school work will be distracted later when playing outside, worrying about what the teacher will say about the homework.

When the Kempoka masters the concept of Kiai in training, he or she will have better concentration at home, at work, in school, in every activity. Many people have noticed that young people in Kempo improve their grades, never realizing exactly why. The increased concentration developed by the Kata is the cause.

Aiki: Harmonious Spirit

The second aspect of Ki that one can develop in Kata is Aiki. This word comprises the same two Kanji that Kiai uses, but in the reverse position. Aiki means "harmonious spirit." Whereas Kiai is the focus of all personal power into one point for a powerful strike, the concept of Aiki is the blending of one's personal energy with the energy generated by the attacker, usually by throwing or controlling the attacker in some grappling manner.

In this way, the harder a person strikes, the harder the person will be thrown. The beginner does not always understand this because grappling in the Western sense is a matter of hard, physical struggle. But in the methods of Kempo Jujutsu and the Torite of Kempo Karate, a throw or joint lock that one struggles to achieve is simply a poor technique.

When a person attacks, he or she cannot help but generate energy. To strike or grapple, the attacker must generate force. By properly applying

Aiki, the defender brings the force into harmony, moving in a way that does not resist the energy but encourages it to continue its course. At some point, the Kempoka leads the assailant beyond the assailant's ability to control both the energy of the attack and the additional energy of the defender. At this point, the defender can throw or lock the opponent, or turn the energy back on the opponent, which will throw the attacker in a reverse manner.

Aiki teaches that it is better to move with, that is, cooperate with, the movements of an attacker rather than go against him or her. When force meets force, the defender will be hurt even in winning the fight, but with Aiki it is possible to defend without being injured. When carried to its highest level, it is possible to win without hurting the antagonist. The Kempoka learns that in life it is better to harmonize with people than to compete with them.

Yoki: Positive Spirit

The last application of Ki that one can develop in Kata is Yoki, which means "positive spirit" or "liveliness." This principle gives a martial artist the ability to overpower and outlast an attacker, or even multiple attackers, by providing the endless energy of Ki.

In a fight, the participants expend a lot of energy in a short time. Endurance is a significant factor, one that often determines the winner in a boxing match. In a real-life struggle, the draw on energy is even greater. If one can train to maintain calm and keep breathing under control, he or she can draw on the Ki for the energy necessary to handle any situation.

Finally, Yoki teaches the Kempoka to look for the positive side of life. In martial-arts practice, some activities challenge the physical and mental capabilities of the Kempoka. It is through these challenges that the student improves. Without challenges, the martial artist does not become stronger, faster, smarter, or better. Kempo improves the student by the challenges it presents.

A good student of Kempo comes to look at life the same way. The challenges of life make us stronger and better people if we meet them the same way we meet challenges in the Dojo. No matter what the challenge, it contains a lesson that can help us become better people if we maintain a positive spirit.

Thus in Kata we develop Ki as Kiai, focused energy; Aiki, blended energy; and Yoki, endless energy. These three aspects are not only fighting principles but also principles of life that enrich our daily existence, allowing us to have a happier life.

The most esoteric aspect about Ki and its development through Kata is the oneness and awareness that the Kempoka develops through the practice. The Kempo practitioner begins to realize through focus on Ki in Kata practice that he or she has a strength, an energy inside. The Kempoka becomes aware, by feeling it, that this Ki is of a spiritual nature.

Once the Kempoka senses his or her individual Ki and realizes how powerful it is, he or she begins to wonder where this great strength comes from and how so much of it could be inside a mortal frame. This leads the Kempoka to the feeling that the Ki within is connected to a greater source without. The move from sensing a personal Ki to the feeling of what could be called the Universal Ki is the spiritual journey.

Eventually, each Kata takes on the feeling of an immersion within this Universal Ki. The Kempoka finds the oneness with the Ultimate and comes to know through the stillness of movement the Absolute. Many Christian martial artists have found a closer relationship to God through this practice of Kempo. They find in each Kata a greater sense of peace and union with the Almighty.

Kata at its highest level is a form of moving meditation that opens students of Kempo to the experience of their spiritual nature and the source of that spirit. This occurs as students develop understanding of the fighting principle of Ki and its three manifestations in actual self-defense: Kiai, Aiki, and Yoki. Through this heightened perception of Ki, the Kempoka realizes the union of the individual Ki and the Universal Ki.

Kaihi

Dodging is an important part of taisabaki. But the best Japanese word for dodging, as it applies to the martial arts, is *kaihi*. This very descriptive term allows the Kempoka who fully understands its meaning a greater depth of comprehension of the nature and importance of dodging, as it relates to combat.

Kai means "go around," which is the best advice for someone faced with either a budding confrontation or an all-out assault. Many fights can be avoided by "going around" the threat, deflecting the potential confrontation through a disinclination to combat the adversary. When an attack has been launched, rather than meeting the force of the attack head on, the best avenue of movement is to go around the offending limb. If someone throws a punch at your face, slide to the outside of the arm, so that the punch misses you completely. This way, you don't risk the person smashing into you.

Some martial artists of certain styles feel they can take a punch anywhere on the body without ill effect. While this is a very impressive ability, most masters of those styles tell their students to dodge. Why? Because dodging works against any attack, be it knife, stick, or hand. It works against kicks, too. And if you find ever yourself in front of a moving car, dodging can keep you from being hurt. Indeed, there are times when "going around" is the only sensible thing to do. The second part of the word, *hi*, means "to ward off," which, unlike dodging, suggests physical contact. Usually warding off, also called blocking, is a function of the hand or arm, but it can also be done with the leg or foot. In any case, the point of blocking is not to avoid an attack, as is done through dodging, but to deflect it, which of course gains a measure of safety. A Kempoka never counts solely on dodging or on blocking but concentrates on both: If a block misses, the body has dodged out of the way; if a dodge fails, the block has deflected the attack.

VISUALIZATION

As Kempoka practice Kata, they are taught that to be effective they must develop the skill known as visualization. Modern psychologists have examined this method of practice and found it valuable in developing everything from a positive attitude to a winning technique in a physical skill.

In the martial arts, visualization is extremely important because a person cannot go out and have actual fights each day. How is it, then, that a person can develop great martial-arts skill without fighting? The answer is Kata. And how can Kata, which includes no fighting, develop the ability to win in battle? The answer is visualization, which can be written in three ways: Shingan, Shinsho, Shinzo.

Shingan: The Mind's Eye

The three words just mentioned give us a guideline on how to develop our visualization. It begins with Shingan, which means "the mind's eye." The beginning Kempoka practicing Kata must visualize the attackers and their attacks as he or she goes through the movements of the form. The Kempoka usually sees this in the mind, using imagination to create the visuals of the Kata.

The martial artist can also use visualization out in the world. Good instructors will ask their students to imagine themselves in various situations. Suppose you were walking down the street and someone jumped out at you from an alley. What would you do if someone attacked you as you were getting in your car?

In Kata, as the person imagines the different attacks that might occur, he or she physically goes through the moves it would take to deal with such an assault. Some forms of martial arts use prearranged Kata. Thus instructors must teach specific visualizations so that their students can develop the necessary skills.

Other styles of martial arts, including certain styles of Kempo, teach a method of freestyle Kata. Students imagine what the attacks are and then move spontaneously to deal with them. According to history, freestyle Kata practice was the method of training for real combat. By picturing multiple attackers and then moving to defend against them, a person learns how to move instinctively, a necessary skill for self-defense. Shingan is seeing the movements in the mind and then performing the moves that meet the visualized scenario.

Shinsho: 3-D Image

But this is just the beginning. Next, the Kempoka wants to develop Shinsho, which means "mental image." Now, however, the student creates a three-dimensional picture. Like the hologram in the Star Trek shows, the Kempoka "sees" the surrounding attackers, allowing greater realism in training.

Because only in Kata can the martial artist perform techniques full out, it is essential that the practitioner have a realistic target. One can accomplish this only through proper visualization. Seeing the attackers, the Kempoka punches, kicks, and strikes legitimate nerve centers, as he or she would in actual self-defense. The visualization must be so accurate that it is no different from having real people in the area.

Kata practice now becomes valid. Kata is like having a real fight, except that no one gets hurt. With good visualization, the body and mind experience the same sensation they would in a real battle, but without the danger or the gratuitous development of fighting for fun, as in competitive martial art.

The mind does not distinguish between a well-visualized Kata and an actual fight. The Kempo practitioner thus gains real self-defense experience without having to fight or harm a human being. Keep in mind that the Shaolin monks and the famous ancient Okinawan fighters developed their great fighting skill through Kata. Neither of these groups of warriors believed in mock competitive fighting. They practiced only Kata.

Shinzo: Other Senses

We can take one additional step with visualization, represented by the term Shinzo, which also translates as "mental image." But now the Kempoka adds other sensory perceptions to the "visualizations." As the martial artist practices the Kata, he or she now feels hands grab the wrists or shoulders, feels his or her body encircled in bear hugs, and hears footsteps coming up from behind. In real-life combat, any number of things can save your life. One should practice these in Kata.

When the sun is behind a person, a shadow leads. Seeing a shadow approaching swiftly from behind may be enough warning to save your life if you are perceptive enough to notice it. Reflections in a store window, in a mirror in a restaurant, or in the glass door of the refrigerated area of a convenience store may be the warning that saves your life. You can practice with these minute warnings in Kata.

The idea of Shinzo is to construct with your imagination the most realistic scenario you can visualize. Moving in this imaginary world helps you develop the skill you will need in real-life self-defense. According to psychologists, many people underestimate the power of visualization. When you need to learn how to face a situation, from self-defense to public speaking, you need only imagine the event occurring and your going through the motions of dealing with it. Doing this exercise will prepare you to deal with the situation.

This is what Kata does to prepare a person for self-defense. Yet the Kata is only as good as the sense of visualization with which one performs it. Kata is excellent physical training, yet it becomes mental training as well through the process of visualization. Although Shingan, Shinsho, and Shinzo all are translated as "visualization," the ideas set forth allow them to be reminders of the depth of visualization that the Kempoka seeks.

BUNKAI: ANALYSIS

One of the most important aspect of martial-arts training is Bunkai, or analysis. When a person begins practicing Kempo, he or she learns that each move can have many meanings. These meanings are only as vast as the Kempoka's understanding, which often depends on having a good instructor.

I have on many occasions been approached by someone who has trained in another style and is seeking help in interpreting the moves of prearranged Kata. Not wanting to contradict the teachings of the student's instructor, I asked first about the instructor's interpretation. Every move in a Kata should have a practical application. If it does not, it has no reason to be there. In truth, every move that a Kempoka learns has multiple meanings, which are determined by what he or she has visualized. A movement at long range will have a vastly different interpretation from the same movement at medium or close range.

A good example is the reverse knife hand, which begins with the left hand held across the body with the palm toward the right ear. The martial artist then extends the arm out away from the body, with the palm rotating down. At long range, this can be a block to the attacking arm of an assailant. At medium range, this can be a strike to the neck of an assailant. At close range, this can be a throw, with the arm passing across the chest of the attacker, knocking the attacker over the left leg, which the practitioner moves into position behind the attacker's legs. Thus the same move has three different uses.

In Kata, the Kempoka should constantly consider these Bunkai as he or she goes through the moves, visualizing rhythm, timing, and distancing. Analysis is not a one-time event, but an ever-changing concept that allows the Kempoka's understanding and knowledge to grow with each practice of the Kata.

Honte: Straightforward Meaning

The Kempo practitioner should develop and use the Bunkai process in five distinct interpretations. The first is the most direct interpretation, the straightforward meaning of each move. This is called the Honte, the "regular skill." In this, a straight-ahead punch is just that, a punch that shoots straight forward and strikes the attacker.

Gyakute: Backward Motion

Next is the Gyakute, the "reverse skill." This skill uses the movement in a manner that takes it backward through the motion of its original pattern. For example, a punch usually starts at the hip and moves straight forward to strike an attacker. The same movement done in reverse brings the fist back into place at the hip, which means that the elbow sticks out behind the defender. Thus the Gyakute of a punch is a back elbow strike, used to strike someone behind the defender.

Kakushite: Hidden Skills

Third are Kakushite, literally "hidden skills." What appear to be intermediate positions in many techniques are actually hidden strikes, joint locks, breaking techniques, and even throws. These hidden skills are not evident without a great deal of understanding and practice, but most of all they require Bunkai.

A good Kempoka understands that wasted movements do not exist in Kempo; thus the flick of a finger should have meaning. An example of a Kakushite is the loading movement for the reverse knife hand. To prepare a strike with the left knife hand, one brings the left hand into position beside the right ear, while the right hand points straight ahead underneath the left arm. When one throws the reverse knife hand, the right hand loads at the side of the body as if one is preparing it for a thrust.

Yet if an attacker is close, the load for the reverse knife hand with the left arm is actually a spear hand thrust with the right hand. This is the hidden technique, a move totally unexpected by most people yet quite evident to the Kempo practitioner who has mastered the concept of Kakushite. As the Kempoka goes through each move in the practice of Kata, he or she evaluates the preliminary movement for what it could be if the distancing in a battle were to change suddenly.

Hente: Changing Skill

The next aspect of Bunkai is Hente, literally the "changing skill." If fighting were an exact science, if people did not deviate from set patterns, it would be possible to teach a series of techniques that would include the ideal response to every action of an opponent. Students would learn that if an opponent does A, they should do B. In fact, many poorly trained individuals believe this kind of learning is sufficient. They collect all the Waza they can to deal with the situations they feel might occur in a fight.

In real life, however, anything can happen. When a person has learned some basic Waza, he or she should then learn how to change these basic skills into others that can meet any situation. One may know only a handful of techniques, but with the Bunkai of Hente he or she will be able to modify them to meet many possibilities.

Some examples of Hente, also known in some martial arts as Henka, follow. Let us say that a Kempoka learns to block a thrust with a left block and then to right punch into the ribs of the opponent. But let us say that upon being blocked, the opponent pulls the arm in to protect the ribs. Following the idea of Hente, the Kempoka would simply change the path of the punch to strike the next available target.

Suppose a Kempoka is taught to use a hip throw on someone who throws a punch and brings the feet together. The Kempoka then faces an attacker who throws the punch but leaves the right foot back. The Kempoka would simply adjust his or her footwork to meet the situation, thus making use of the idea of Hente.

It is Hente (Henka) that produced the rich diversity of throws from Kempo Jujutsu and other Jujutsu systems, including Aikido and Judo. These include hip throws performed with the arm around the waist, across the shoulder blades at an angle, around the neck, grabbing the belt, holding one arm, and grasping the lapel. All these hip throws are variations, Henka, created by using the Hente, the "changing skill."

Sutemite: Sacrifice Skills

The fifth interpretation in Bunkai involves the Sutemite, which literally means "sacrifice skills." These movements seem to place the Kempoka in a weakened or vulnerable position but allow him or her to deliver a surprise technique against the opponent. The most obvious sacrifice, which nearly everyone has seen in either movies or television shows, is the throw in which a person places the foot against the abdomen of an attacker and then falls to his or her back. The falling is the sacrifice, which ends up throwing the attacker head over heels beyond the defender.

Occasionally, a Kempoka might slide to the ground to deliver a kick to the legs or abdomen of an attacker. Kempoka use sacrifice techniques sparingly because unless they work, the defender is in a poor position to continue a defense. But when one can deliver it with absolute surprise, the technique tends to be devastating.

Bunkai is considered the most important aspect of Kata training because it provides the opportunity for students to learn on their own. At first, an instructor must give the students Oyo, applications, for the movements they are learning and using in their Kata. The instructor does this to teach the student the process of Bunkai. The goal of a good Kempo instructor is to teach students how to Bunkai, how to analyze movements, how to understand what they can and cannot use in a real-life situation.

In this way, the art of Kempo keeps evolving and improving to meet the needs of a changing society. Techniques designed to work against an opponent clad in traditional Japanese armor have little meaning today, but one might use a modified form of such movements to battle someone in a bulletproof vest or heavy winter coat.

Movements never change. Humans are basically the same as they were two thousand years ago. Only their societies have changed. Techniques that mainm and kill must be modified so that people can defend themselves without going to prison, but most techniques will stay basically the same.

For example, a simple wristlock is today usually taught as a method of taking a person to the ground and then controlling him or her. Originally, however, the wristlock was a devastating wrist counter designed to destroy the wrist so that the person could not hold a sword or make a fist. During the modern era, martial-arts instructors have modified the skill to meet the needs of today's self-defense rather than the combat situation of feudal Japan. Good Kempo instructors, however, know the necessity of teaching all skills, for no one knows when he or she will be thrust into a life-threatening situation.

Part of Bunkai is the ability to change techniques from soft to hard, from control to break, from stunning to killing, according to the situation. Kempo has correctly been called the deadliest of all martial arts. Although most martial arts have been modified to such a degree that they no longer retain their combat origins, Kempo, through the process of Bunkai, maintains all its skills.

Through study of Honte, Gyakute, Kakushite, Hente, and Sutemite, the Kempoka can maintain all the real skills of Kempo. Through Kata and proper visualization, a Kempoka can safely practice the most destructive skills of Kempo. Through the process of Bunkai, the practitioner can develop all the skills necessary for survival. Kempo is the most effective of all the martial arts for true self-defense because of the proper application of Bunkai to Kata.

Teaching
Kempo

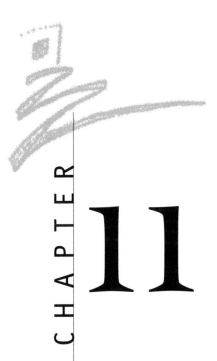

T he Kempoka can continue his or her education by choosing a Soke, a headmaster, to work with. The Soke has a depth of experience and shares the knowledge at a school, called a Dojo.

SOKE: THE HEADMASTER

The head of a system of martial arts may be known by many different names. The title with the most prestige and history is the term pronounced in Japanese as Soke. Most Japanese and Okinawan masters of traditional martial-arts systems use this title.

The term originated in China. Through the lineage of Zen, it connects to the history of the martial arts. It seems that after Bodhidharma founded the Zen sect of Buddhism, the headmastery of the faith passed through five patriarchs, listed here with the Chinese name preceding the Japanese pronunciation.

Bodhidharma, Daruma

Huike, Eka

Seng tsan, Sosan

Tao shin, Doshin

Hung jen, Gunin

Hui neng, Sokei Eno

TENSHIN SHO

According to Donn Draeger, one of the first Occidentals to study classical martial arts in Japan, the original martial arts began with a divine illumination, known in the Orient, particularly in Japan, as a Tenshin Sho. The martial arts were not just fighting skills for survival, though they certainly were those. More important to those who practiced them, they were ways of life.

To be true to the name, a martial art must include three elements. The first is that a martial art must be concerned with real combat—not sport, not competition, not egotistical fighting, but real struggle, whether on a personal basis or in war. The skills must be real. As martial arts develop into sports, whether as fighting forms or artistic expressions, they begin to adopt unrealistic methods of movement that have no value in genuine combat. This means that they cease being martial arts and become something else.

The second aspect of a true martial art is artistic expression. The relevant term here is Jutsu, meaning "art" and referring to the fact that practitioners internalize the skill to produce creativity in motion. This creativity is the only way martial-arts skills can be truly effective. A person who merely copies others finds it almost impossible to develop workable skills in self-defense. A martial artist must practice to the point where the skill becomes his or her own. The practitioner moves in a unique, individual way that incorporates the knowledge and skill of his or her master.

Watch two Kempoka who have trained under the same master. They can perform the same skill, but you will notice a slight difference between the performances. Neither is wrong. Each does it his or her way, from within. A good Kempo teacher shows students the way to do something, tells them why he or she does it that way, and then lets them discover for themselves how to do it. Learning how to perform a technique is always a matter of self-exploration and self-discovery. Too much instruction is as harmful as too little.

Thus teachers instructed people in a martial art and expected them to discover the personal art within themselves. This second level of development in the true martial arts leads to the third, the development of Ki.

As Ki empowers all true martial arts, so too it starts the Kempoka on the spiritual journey that is the ultimate destination of true martial-arts training. The final level of martial-arts training is spiritual enlightenment. If a martial art does not seek this aspect for its practitioners, it is not a classical, or real, martial art.

Enlightenment can be a confusing concept. It is not about doctrine, dogma, or religion; it is about experience. Look at the word: *en·light·en·ment.*

Enlightenment is about looking beyond the phenomenal world to see the essence it comes from. All faiths speak of the light, yet many stop short of teaching their adherents to strive to see the light. Many religions, established in the light, have retreated into darkness, teaching their participants to believe in the light rather than to bathe in it.

The martial arts are not about religion. Though originally developed by Buddhist monks, they have spread to Taoist, Shintoists, Christians, Muslims, Jews, and people of many other faiths. Martial arts generally do not seek to convert people but merely to instruct them to "see." What they do with what they see is always up to them.

To be worthy of the title Soke, a person must have had a spiritual experience in which he or she saw the light. The understanding a person gained from that experience gave rise to the flow of the individual's martial art. On a technical level the art looked the same, for in truth the human body can only do so much in movement for combat or survival. But the way the martial-arts master taught it, the philosophy behind it, grew from that person's experience.

A Tenshin Sho was a personal experience. A master would tell the story of the experience but often leave out certain aspects, revealing them only to special disciples. The experience changed the master's life. The person who had not been of a spiritual nature developed spiritually. The master who had already been spiritual became more so.

Yet masters maintained an earthiness, for they needed to pass on their new, spiritually gained wisdom to their students. Some individuals did not plan to do the martial arts as a lifetime endeavor, but ended up dedicating their whole lives to the spreading of their art, simply because of the Tenshin Sho.

When masters experience an awakening, which is what the experience really is, they feel compelled to put the encounter into words. They often cannot truly express what happened. The limitation of the written or spoken

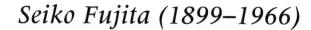

Seiko Fujita (1899–1966)

Known more prominently for his connection as the last master of Koga Ryu Ninjutsu, Seiko Fujita was also the headmaster of Sato Ryu Kempo. During his life, he taught many students and befriended the Okinawan martial arts master, Choki Motobu. Fujita encouraged his Japanese students to study the Okinawan martial arts, seeking a greater degree of knowledge and skill from the synthesis of the two countries' martial arts.

Fujita sought to practice from the foundation of Olympic training of Japanese athletes. He specialized in little-known aspects of kempo training, such as *karumijutsu* (body lightening art), *hichojutsu* (jumping and climbing art), and *suieijutsu* (combat swimming art). Through his teachings, these esoteric forms of training have passed down to modern times. It is believed Fujita instructed James Masayoshi Mitose during their time within the entourage of Choki Motobu.

word leads to the esoteric teachings of the martial arts, as masters struggle with the "truth" of their experience.

Many masters express the Tenshin Sho in the title of their Ryu. Hidden within the name is the light they saw, as they can best explain it in frail human terms. Masters devote the rest of their lives to expressing the inexpressible, to describing the infinite spirit to the finite minds of their students.

Thus a person who is truly a Soke of a genuine Ryu has had a divine experience that was life changing and mind expanding. This experience is generally what impelled the person to teach the martial arts and establish a Ryu, or system. The true Soke is one who has seen and knows an experience. Moreover, the Soke wants all students, and in essence, all the world to know. This is the true Soke, the true "head of the house," one who wants all to see the light.

KENSHO

Kensho means a "seeing of the light." In the same way that all members of a church seek the same faith, so the members of a Ryu seek to experience the same light. Just as a minister is called to head the church, the Soke is called to head the Ryu.

We noted earlier that a Soke has had a Tenshin Sho, an experience of seeing a divine illumination. What then, many ask, can the regular student of Kempo experience? The student may not see an earth-shattering or life-changing event but still wants to make the spiritual journey that the Soke has taken. What can a Deshi, a student, of Kempo expect on a spiritual level?

This relevant question was answered hundreds of years ago when the first Chugoku Kempo masters wanted their students to grow spiritually. The answer has been passed down from generation to generation, from

China to Japan, from Okinawa to America. What a student is striving for is a Kensho.

After having an experience, the Soke expressed it as a philosophy, which was an attempt to express the light. Students who enter a Ryu and hear the teachings of the philosophy stay because it appeals to them. It speaks to their hearts. Through listening to the teachings, they become closer to the experience that the Soke originally had.

Yet in the martial arts, physical training is intricately linked with spiritual development. Students thus realize that they can grow in the same way as the Soke did by practicing with the dedication and attitude of the Soke.

The light is there for all to see. It is not hidden. People who have seen the light realize this and wonder why it took so long for them to see it. They wonder why not everyone can see it. The Soke, upon achieving an awakening, immediately desires it for all students of the Ryu. The Soke wants to have as many students as possible, not just for the sake of the Ryu, but for the sake of the individuals who will "see" the light.

When a student achieves a Kensho, an awakening, he or she experiences the joy of the light. The person then wants to share this joy with others, realizing that he or she accomplished the goal through martial-arts training. The person seeks to bring others to his or her school, hoping that new students will see the light as well.

A Ryu is not a cult. It does not teach a set of doctrines that all must embrace for the benefit of the group and to the detriment of the individual. Rather, a Ryu allows people to have their own lives and express their enlightenment as they see fit. Most Christian martial artists who experience a Kensho during martial-arts training become deeper, more devout Christians. Those of other faiths similarly become more pious. James Masayoshi Mitose became a Christian minister and spoke about the teachings of Buddha that coincided with those of Christ.

The seeing of the light frees students to express themselves as they choose. The Soke does not control or manipulate students but is available to counsel and advise them when the need arises. The Soke hopes that a mature development of the sprit will accompany the Kensho so that students continue to progress in life—living the philosophy of the Ryu, enjoying the fellowship of other students, and helping to teach the martial arts.

RYUHA

Sometime between the 9th century and the 12th century the concept of Ryu developed in Japan. A Ryu was a martial-arts school that taught the fighting style and philosophy of a certain individual. Bushi or Samurai who had fought in the wars of Japan and developed exceptional skills that allowed them to survive generally founded these schools. These warriors organized their skills into some kind of curriculum. They added a philosophical base, which they usually expressed in the religious terms of their particular faith. For the most part, however, they did not force their religion on their students. They called merely for an increase in spiritual awareness and turned what previously had been a loose body of knowledge into a Ryuha, a school of thought with the martial arts as its foundation.

The Shodai, or founder, of a school established it not with the idea of becoming famous or wealthy but out of a desire to pass on to his students what he had learned. When the Ryu were first developed, they were kept secret and made available only to personal family members, or the clan. The Soke of the Ryu wanted to make sure that members of his family were secure in their ability to defend themselves and that the clan was strong enough to maintain its land and possessions.

Eventually, alliances developed among clans, which meant that the best masters among them taught the warriors who would be protecting their land. Yet regardless of how few one's sons and daughters, or how many nephews, cousins, or paid warriors a Soke taught, he treated all his students as family.

Although the foundation of many of the martial arts was Zen and others were more associated with Mikkyo (Tantric Buddhism), the personal beliefs of the Soke were generally of a more comprehensive nature. Japanese of all religions tended to have a strong Shinto base. Thus when students sat at the foot of a Soke to learn martial arts, they received a broad philosophical foundation, learning aspects of Shinto, Dokyo (Taoism), Confucianism, Buddhism, along with the personal experience of the Soke.

The Ryuha, the actual school of thought of a Soke, was generally based on personal experience in combat and a religious occurrence that solidified the experience into a philosophical statement from which the Soke taught. This philosophical base formed both the moral foundation and the fighting concept of the Ryu.

Although the art did not change physically, strategically it underwent a major metamorphosis. How things were done remained the same, but the why of it became based on the Soke's testimonial. It was certain that the Soke was right, first, because he was alive. He had combat experience, had faced the shadow of death and survived.

The second reason a Soke was believed to be right was that the only legitimate reason for founding a Ryu was a divine inspiration. The history of the martial arts includes many stories of warriors gaining religious insight from divine messengers and then creating their schools. In some cases, the visitation was from an angelic being. In others, an ancestor or great warrior from the past would visit. In still others, a living monk would arrive and teach a great spiritual insight to the warrior.

Regardless, the Soke was seen as right because of his great life experience, religious insight, and good heart. The Soke taught for the benefit of his students. If he did not care if others lived or died, why would he teach? The real Soke wanted to pass the learning on to others for the benefit of those others.

For this reason, after the Soke began teaching people other than their family members, they still ran the Ryu as they would a family. Soke literally means the "head, or master, of a house." The term *ka* at the end of Kempoka is the same character as the *ke* of Soke. *Ka* means "member of the house." In other words, the Soke is the father and the Kempoka are his children. The Soke cares about his children.

The concept of the Ryu as a school of martial arts is a uniquely Japanese institution. Other terms were used for martial-arts groups in China. In that country, a martial art was taught either at a Ssu, temple; Pai, association; or Kuan, school.

Although similar terms were used in Japan, the tradition and teachings of the Soke was called the Ryu. The Ryu might be taught in a Kan, school, on in a group of schools called Kai, an association.

The Ryu was the family, which encompassed anywhere from a few students to hundreds. Some Soke never had more than one small Dojo, preferring to keep the unit small and personal. A few taught for Daimyo, feudal lords, and taught hundreds of warriors who served their master.

Today Soke are found in nearly every country where the Oriental martial arts have taken hold. Some have assumed the title with no formal recognition, others have started Ryu to be the heads of their own organizations, and a few have received a Tenshin Sho in the original manner. These Soke continue to follow the traditions established by the original Japanese masters, who conferred on worthy Okinawan martial-arts masters the title and heritage of the Soke and their Ryu. In turn, as serious and dedicated martial artists from around the world have proved their worth, they have received proper and formal recognition from the Orient to be the Shodai, the founders of their own Ryu, and to lead their systems as Soke of their own martial-arts families.

Kenwa Mabuni (1889–1952)

Mabuni began training at age 13 under two of the greatest martial-arts instructors in Okinawa, Yasutsune Itosu and Kanryo Higashionna. He combined what he had learned from the two masters to form his own style. Mabuni taught in Japan and helped introduce the Okinawan martial art to the mainland.

Mabuni preferred to call his art Kempo Karate. His student Kanyei Uechi took his style back to Okinawa. Shito Ryu Kempo Karate is a complete style, encompassing throwing skills, empty-hand striking, and weaponry.

Mabuni influenced the development of many martial arts, including many of the Kempo systems in the United States. Most styles of Shito Ryu derive from Kenwa Mabuni's style.

DOJO

Many Buddhist temples in the past had a special room known as the way place, which in Japanese is pronounced Dojo. In that room the monks sought to know the way through Zazen, seated meditation.

As time passed and many monks learned Kempo, the room was sometimes used for martial-arts practice, with the monks still seeking the way, even in the midst of their Kempo movements.

When the Buddhist monks shared their religion and their Kempo with lay people, their students became aware of the concept of the Dojo. These students realized that even as they sought to develop their fighting skills so that they could better protect themselves and serve their Daimyo, so too did they seek to follow the way and know the spiritual path of righteousness.

Thus at that point in the past, the Japanese warriors adopted the name Dojo for their martial-arts schools. Some believe the Japanese people to be the most spiritual people in the world. The act of identifying their martial-arts schools with a name that referenced spiritual growth offers some proof of that opinion.

Even in the cities of America, martial-arts schools today are known as Dojo. A Kempo school that derives from a Japanese or Okinawan origin takes pride in the fact that it is a Dojo, not a gymnasium. Whether practicing in a small room in a YMCA, in a dance studio, in the corner of a gym, or in a racquetball court, when the spirit is right, the Kempo class is being held in a Dojo.

The Dojo is not the room or the building; it is the people and the spirit of their endeavor. True Kempoka are people seeking to grow spiritually during this journey we call life. They are martial artists seeking to know the way of peace by practicing the art of war.

A Dojo is a place of self-discovery, a place where people work hard to strip away the veneer of illusions they have created around themselves. The idea of the Dojo is to create a spiritual environment that encourages the Kempoka to seek and search their own spirits, with the idea of discovering their true selves.

A true Kempo school, no matter how rustic or how ornate, must live up to the idea that it is a "way place" where sincere practitioners of the martial arts can enroll on the journey of self-discovery. The Dojo must be a place where Kempoka seek to help the novice along the way, even as they help one another on the same journey. The Dojo should be home.

Kempo has evolved over the years in its purpose and training yet always maintaining the ancient principles on which it was founded. From the Sohei of the 6th century to the Sokes of the 21st Kempo is not merely a study of martial arts and its strikes, thrusts, and kicks, Kempo is a way of life, bringing peace and fulfillment to everyone who chooses to encompass its true meaning.

GLOSSARY

Aikido—Grappling martial art based on Jujutsu founded by Morihei Ueshiba in the 1940s

Aikijujutsu—Ancient system of martial arts reputedly created by Yoshimitsu Minamoto in the 12th century

Aikijutsu—High level of martial spiritual development based on love

Aikite—Harmony hand

Aite—Opponent, in Kempo, more appropriately, partner

Ashigaru—Foot soldiers of the Japanese warriors

Ashisabaki—Foot and leg movement

Bokken—Wooden sword

Bu—Martial, literally "to stop violence"

Bugei—Martial arts, the multiple disciplines of combat including about 50 skills

Bujutsu—Martial art, usually a way of referencing one of the Bugei at a time, sometimes used as a synonym of Bugei

Bunkai—Analysis, or analyzation, used to develop applications of a movement

Busan—Martial creativity

Bushi—Warrior, the highest level of Japanese warrior

Bushi Te—Warrior hand, the skill of the warrior, a secret martial art practiced only by Okinawan warriors in antiquity

Butoku—Martial virtue

Chin na—Chinese grappling skills similar to Jujutsu

Choshi—Rhythm

Chuanfa—Chinese way of pronouncing Kempo, meaning "fist law"

Chugoku—Japanese term for China, literally "middle country"

Daimyo—Feudal lord of Japan

Daito Ryu—System taught by Sokaku Takeda, reputedly founded by Yoshimitsu Minamoto

Dojo—Martial-arts school, literally "way place"

Embu—Martial exercises, two-person method of training

Fudoshin—Immovable mind, imperturbability

Go no Kempo—Strength fist law, used in reference to Okinawan martial arts derived from Shaolin styles

Gogyo—Five elements, used in Taoist philosophy, also used as a basis for martial-arts strategy in the internal styles

Goju Ryu—Okinawan style of martial arts founded by Chojun Miyagi

Goken—Literally "five fists," Japanese term for the five animal forms of Shaolin Chuanfa

Gyakute—Reverse skill

Hakkakkei—Octagon, a principle used by Mitose to teach martial-arts strategy and skill

Hakke Ken—Eight trigrams fist, an internal style of Chinese Kempo, in Chinese pronounced Pa Kua Chuan

Hakutsuru Ken—White-crane fist, a style of Chinese martial art influential to Okinawan martial arts

Haragei—Spiritual arts, centralization, a high-level concept of martial-arts development

Heiho—Literally "soldiers' method," strategy

Henka—Variations, different ways of applying techniques

Hente—Changing skill

Hichojutsu—Leaping and flying art, also used in reference to specialized climbing skills

Himitsu Kempo—Secret fist law, a special form of martial arts taught in the temples of Japan

Ho—Law, method, way; the Japanese word for the Dharma of Buddhist philosophy

Honshin—Right mind, the ability to make good decisions

Honte—Regular skill

Hung Chia—A southern style of Chinese Kempo based on Shaolin martial arts, influential in several Okinawan Karate styles

Hyomen Dome—Surface stopping, a principle of training focus in Kempo

Hyomen Hakai—Surface destruction, a principle of Kempo self-defense focus causing exterior damage

Hyoshi—Timing

I Chuan—Will boxing, a Chinese style of martial arts studied by Chojun Miyagi, a combination of Tai Chi, Hsing I, and Pa Kua

Ikite—The relaxed hand, principle of In

Ikken Hissatsu—Literally "one fist, certain death," the ultimate principle of Okinawan striking arts

In Yo—Japanese pronunciation of Yin Yang, a principle of the universe applied to martial-arts strategy

Jigen Ryu Bujutsu—The martial arts of the Satsuma Samurai who ruled Okinawa from 1609 to 1868, studied by several Okinawan warriors

Jisamurai—Farmer-warriors of Japan who lived in the rural areas and farmed when not soldiering

Jiyu Kata—Freestyle form, the original method of form training

Ju no Kempo—Gentle fist law, used in reference to Chinese internal systems and Jujutsu as they influenced the Okinawan arts

Judo—System of martial arts based on Jujutsu and founded by Jigoro Kano in 1882

Jujutsu—Japanese empty-hand martial arts, a term coined around the 16th century

Kaihi—Dodging

Kakushite—Hidden skill

Kamae—Posture, used in reference to whole-body attitude

Kamite—Literally "divine hand," an Okinawan reference to the belief that the martial arts are divinely inspired

Kanji—Chinese characters used by the Japanese as their written language

Karate—Empty hand, the term for Okinawan martial arts coined by Chomo Hanashiro in 1903 and adopted for general use by a board of Okinawan masters in 1936

Karumijutsu—Body-lightening art, a secret martial skill taught as part of the Bugei curriculum in traditional systems

Kata—Form, a method of performing skills in a continuous manner

Katana—Sword, specifically used in reference to the long sword carried by the Samurai

Katsute—Resuscitation hand

Keage—Kick up

Kei I—Literally "form will," an internal Chinese form of Kempo, pronounced in Chinese as Hsing I

Keiko—Practice, literally "think of the old"

4473

Kekomi—Kick through

Kempo—Fist law, sometimes translated as "boxing" or "martial arts," a method of martial arts that emphasizes self-defense and realism

Kempoka—Person who practices Kempo

Kendo—Literally "way of the sword," coined to refer to a sport developed around bamboo swords and armor

Kenjutsu—Sword art, the combat skill of fighting with live blades

Kensho—Seeing the light, spiritual insight

Kenshojutsu—Japanese term meaning "fist-palm art," the original form of Shaolin martial art

Keri—Kick

Ki—Spirit, energy, internal strength

Ki Shindo—Energy pulse, the devastating power of a Ki strike, which causes internal damage

Kiai—Spirit harmony, unified energy, sometimes a yell

Kiaijutsu—The art of energy unification, which generates great power for throwing or striking

Kihon—Basics, the fundamental techniques of a martial-arts system

Kihon Kumite—Basic sparring, a method of practicing basics with a partner

Kijutsu—Spirit art, used in reference to spiritual development, also applied to healing arts using Ki

Kime—Literally "decisiveness," used in reference to focus, the concept of focusing a strike into a person's body or a throw to its point of completion

Kinsei—Symmetry

Kiyojute Ryu Kempo Bugei—a traditional martial-arts system taught by the author that preserves the most ancient methods of Kempo and the derivatives of Jujutsu, Karate, and Kobujutsu

Kobujutsu—Ancient martial art, usually used in reference to weapons training or auxiliary skills

Kosho Ryu Kempo—The form of Kempo that James Masayoshi Mitose taught in Hawaii, the first form of Kempo taught outside Japan

Kshatriya—Indian warrior caste

Kumite—Usually translated as "sparring" but actually meaning "cooperative hand," a method of training with a partner

Kyusho—Vital points, the points on the body most vulnerable to injury from striking, including nerves, blood vessels, and body cavities

Maai—Distancing

Makiwari—Literally "wrapped rope," a striking post developed by the Okinawans to condition their hands for self-defense

Mudansha—Students of the martial arts who do not yet hold a black belt

Mukei—No form, a term used for freestyle Kata

Mushin—No mind, keeping extraneous thoughts out of the mind so that spontaneous actions may occur

Nagare—Flow, fluidity

Naginata—A Japanese halberd, used by foot soldiers and favored by many warrior monks

Naibu Hakai—Inner destruction, the principle of Kempo self-defense based on causing interior damage

Ninjutsu—Stealth art, a skill of espionage that teaches specialized techniques of camouflage, methods of entry and extrication, and other surveillance ideas

Odori Te—Literally "dancing hand," a method of training used in advanced Okinawan martial arts, little practiced outside Okinawa

Okuden—Inner "heart" tradition, the most secret teachings of a traditional martial-arts system

Oyo—Applications of a movement forming the various techniques of the martial arts

Renshu—Literally "polish training," another word for practice with the idea of improving skills through repetition

Renzoku Ken—Continuous fist, a term used for combining techniques in a fluid, incessant manner to make an inexorable self-defense skill

Ritsudo—Rhythmic movement

Ryu—System, tradition, school, in this context, of a martial art

Ryuki—The flow of energy, a principle used in performing Renzoku Ken and in blending with an attacker

Samurai—General term for the Japanese warrior

Sato Ryu—A system of Kempo practiced by Seiko Fujita, believed to have been founded in the 12th century

Seiho—Literally "method for putting right," a Japanese method of healing connected to Kempo

Seite—The living hand, keeping spirit in the entire body

Senshin—"Mainly mind," undivided attention, singleness of purpose, concentration

Shaolinssu—The young forest temple, reputedly the birthplace of Kempo, where Bodhidharma developed both Zen and the forerunner of the martial arts

Shih Pa Lo Han Sho—Literally "the 18 hands of an enlightened man," the exercise set reputedly developed by Bodhidharma

Shin—Mind

Shin Shin—Mind and body

Shinai—The bamboo sword used in Kendo and as a means of discipline in many Japanese Dojo

Shingan—Mind's eye

Shinite—The active hand, principle of Yo

Shinken—Literally "divine fist," a term used in Japan in reference to the divine origin of the martial arts

Shinsho—Mental image

Shinzo—Mental image with full sensory perception

Shite—Hand of death

Shorin Ryu—The name of a branch of Okinawan Karate, of which there are many divisions, purportedly derived from Chinese Shorinji Kempo

Shorinji—Japanese pronunciation of the Shaolinssu, young forest temple

Shugyo—Austere training, a concept of practice in which one works hard to improve oneself physically and spiritually

Sohei—Warrior monks of the Japanese temples specially trained in Himitsu Kempo

Suieijutsu—Swimming art, one of the auxiliary skills taught to Samurai

Sumo—A form of grappling sport, unique to Japan and surrounded by Shinto ritual

Sun Dome—Literally "one-inch stop," a method for training focus and maintaining safety in Okinawan martial-arts practice

Sutemite—Sacrifice skill

Tachi—Stance, the stances of the martial arts

Tai—Body

Tai Chi Chuan—The first internal method of Chinese martial arts, based on Taoist principles and emphasizing natural movement and gentleness

Tai Kyoku Ken—The Japanese way of pronouncing Tai Chi Chuan

Taisabaki—Body movement, applied to all movements or, in some systems, applied only to pivoting

Tameshiwari—Literally "test by breaking," the act of breaking boards and tiles as a way of testing one's strength and skill, associated with Okinawan martial arts in particular

Te—Literally "hand" or "skill," the indigenous term used by the Okinawans for their original martial art

Teawase—Hand facing, a term used in Okinawa for a wrestling match that tested one's strength and skill and in which no strikes were allowed

Tegumi—Hand matching, another term used in Okinawa for a wrestling match similar to Sumo, usually of a friendly nature

Tekken—Iron fist, a principle of fighting directed towards the mastery of vital-point striking

Ten Myaku—Literally "point blood vessel," known in Chinese as Dim Mak

Tengu—An angelic being in Japanese legend reportedly taught advanced skills to many martial artists

Tenshin Sho—Divine illumination, the source of inspiration from which martial-arts masters found their Ryu

Tesabaki—Hand movements

To—The sword of Kempo

Tode—Literally "Tang hand," referring to the Chinese influence in Okinawa, can also be pronounced Karate

Torite—Taking hand, the grappling skills of Okinawan martial arts, can be pronounced Tuite or Toide in the Okinawan dialect

Uchi—Strike

Uchite—Literally "striking hand," the skills of hitting with all bodily weapons of Karate and Kempo

Uke—Block

Vajramushti—Diamond fist, the fighting art practiced by the Indian warrior caste, the Kshatriya, known by Bodhidharma

Wako—Japanese pirates who plied the waters of the Orient, attacking villages, pillaging, and robbing

Waza—Techniques, the skills of the martial arts

Wing Chun—A Chinese form of martial arts derived from Shaolinssu Chuanfa with an emphasis on crane techniques, the original system studied by Bruce Lee

Wu—Chinese word for martial, the same as Japanese Bu

Wu Shu—Chinese pronunciation of Bujutsu, martial art

Wute—Chinese pronunciation of Butoku, martial virtue

Yakusoku Kata—Literally "prearranged form," the method of Kata training that developed during the 20th century as a method for teaching Karate to schoolchildren

Yari—Spear

Yoki—Positive spirit, endless energy

Yudansha—Person who holds a black belt in the martial arts

Zanshin—Awareness, literally "surviving mind" or "remaining mind"

Zazen—Literally "seated meditation"

Zen—Meditation, a form of emptying one's mind so that one can directly experience the world, literally "to show one"

INDEX

ABOUT THE AUTHOR

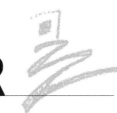

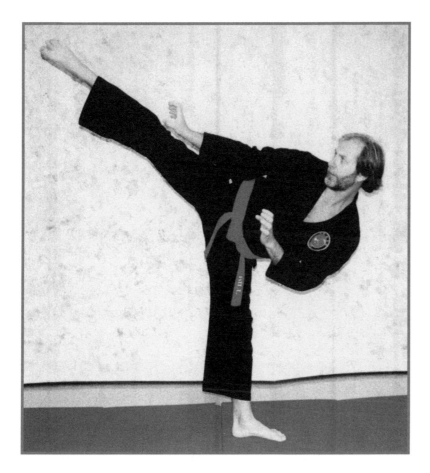

William Durbin, a 30-year student and practitioner of martial arts, has reached the level of Soke, the highest ranking in Kiyojute Kempo. He also holds varying degrees of black belts in judo, karate, taekwondo, and tai chi.

Durbin has a PhD in Oriental philosophy from the University of Oriental Philosophy in Murphy, North Carolina and has made martial arts a lifetime study and passion. He is considered one of the world's foremost authorities and historians on Kempo, the original martial art. Durbin is president of the Christian Martial Arts Association and the Spiritual Martial Arts Research Association. Among his numerous martial arts honors are Presidential Sports Awards for karate and judo. Durbin also has been listed in Who's Who for Karate and American Martial Arts and was chosen as one of the Outstanding Young Men in America.

An ordained minister who emphasizes the spiritual element of martial arts, Durbin has a ministry in Frankfort, Kentucky, where he resides with his wife, Carol.

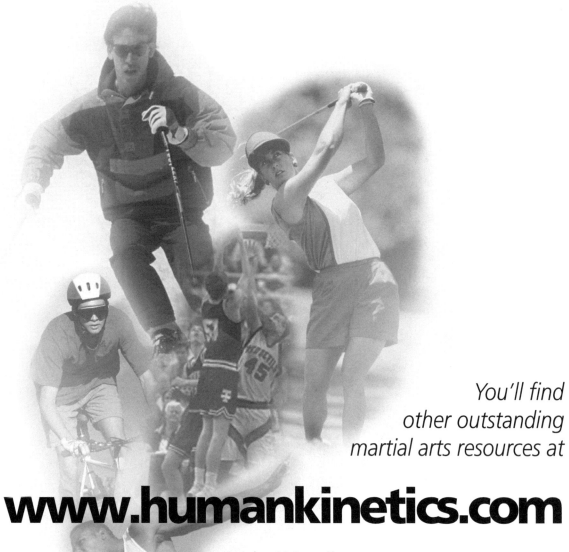